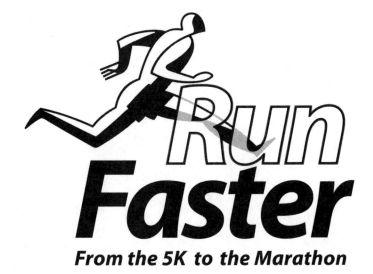

Run Faster

From the 5K to the Marathon

BROADWAY BOOKS   NEW YORK

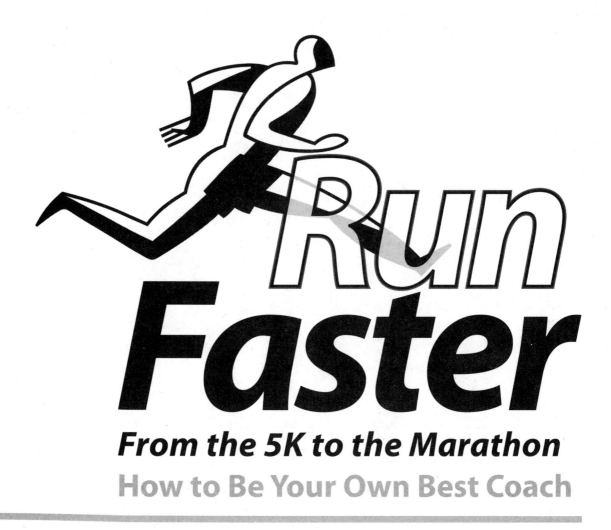

Run Faster

From the 5K to the Marathon

How to Be Your Own Best Coach

Brad Hudson and Matt Fitzgerald

To the Athletes

PUBLISHED BY BROADWAY BOOKS

Published in the United States by Broadway Books, an imprint
of The Doubleday Publishing Group, a division of Random
House, Inc., New York.
www.broadwaybooks.com

BROADWAY BOOKS and its logo, a letter B
bisected on the diagonal, are trademarks of Random House,
Inc.

Book design by Michael Collica

Library of Congress Cataloging-in-Publication Data
Hudson, Brad.
Run faster from the 5K to the marathon : how to be your own
best coach / Brad Hudson and Matt
Fitzgerald.—1st ed.
  p. cm.
1. Running—Training. I. Fitzgerald, Matt. II. Title.
GV1061.5.H83 2008
796.42'4–dc22   2007040944

ISBN 978-0-7679-2822-9

PRINTED IN THE UNITED STATES OF AMERICA

10 9 8 7 6 5 4 3 2

First Edition

Contents

Acknowledgments

Although only two names appear on the cover, this book wouldn't be what it is without vital contributions from the following people, to whom we offer our most heartfelt thanks: Jo Ankier, Jonathon Beverly, Nic Bideau, Bill Bowerman, Casey Burchill, Renato Canova, James Carney, Stacy Creamer, Alan Culpepper, Shayne Culpepper, Bill Dellinger, Donavon Guyot, Jason Hartmann, Lucinda Hull, Christy Johnson, Jeff Johnson, Weldon Johnson, Linda Konner, Megan Lewis, Kelly Liljeblad, Dathan Ritzenhein, Kalin Ritzenhein, Stephanie Rothstein, Victor Sailor, Sarah Schwald, Andy Smith, Sarah Toland, Edwardo Torres, Jorge Torres, Alison Wade, Toby Warden, Mark Wetmore, and Mary Wittenberg.

Foreword

Congratulations. By purchasing this book you are taking advantage of a remarkable opportunity: to learn not just to coach yourself but to coach yourself the way Brad Hudson would if you were a world-class runner under his care. What sets Brad's program apart is its responsiveness to the individual. Rather than relying on cookie-cutter regimens with weeks of prescribed mileage and workouts set in stone, Brad sees how a runner is responding to the training before he decides what the next step should be. And now, armed with the information between these covers, you'll be able to make similar assessments for yourself. The best runner is an educated runner.

Here at New York Road Runners we believe in changing the world for the better, and enriching and enhancing the lives of individuals of all ages and abilities through running. Our efforts range from organizing weekly local races for thousands of runners, to our NYRR Foundation programs, which currently bring running and fitness to more than forty thousand schoolchildren every day in New York City and beyond. We attempt to win people over to the benefits of running—person by person. We know how good running is for people in so many ways. We also know the compelling satisfaction that improvement in running brings. I am happy for you that, with this book, you are on the road to such improvement and satisfaction.

Running is hard. No question about it. It gets easier as one gets fitter, and it also gets to be more fun. This is true for all people—from the very best in the world to the rest of us. The best in the world, like American star Dathan Ritzenhein, Central Park 10K record holder and member of the USA Olympic Marathon team headed to Beijing, are extra talented and work really hard, but they also have some advantages over mere mortals like the rest of us. Some have world-class coaches to support them in their efforts to get fitter and faster. Dathan and his teammates are especially fortunate. They have the benefit of the attention and effort of one of the smartest, hardest-working, most intense coaches in the business, a young man who learned by doing and studying. Coach Brad Hudson leaves no stone unturned in his quest to help his athletes thrive. He's part engineer, part mathematician, part scientist, and part psychologist. Brad is one of those people who pours his heart and soul and mind into what he does. Lucky for our sport, Brad has chosen to coach long-distance running. Now, lucky for you, Brad has translated his learning and teachings into lessons and guidance for everyone.

I remember my first chat with Brad well. It was several years ago in a running store in Boulder, Colorado. I had heard much of this young legend in running, and the moment I met him, I was drawn in by his intense passion for coaching his athletes. I barely knew the guy, but he chewed my ear for an hour on the science of coaching and his expectations for Dathan Ritzenhein to ace the marathon at an early age. He was buoyed by the challenge of getting the then injury-prone Ritzenhein to the start line strong and healthy. Working with Dathan, Brad has now done that repeatedly.

He's now taking the show on the road to your home. Good for you. Enjoy the read and the ride. Run smart and hard and enjoy the satisfaction of the journey . . . all the more satisfying with Brad.

I wish you the very best of luck with your training. And I hope we'll see you at a New York Road Runners race sometime soon.

Mary Wittenberg

President & CEO

New York Road Runners

Introduction:
Every Runner Needs (to Be) a Coach

My life as a runner started with an amazing stroke of good luck. When I was 9 years old, I joined a newly created community running program called "Run for Fun" that was based in my New Jersey hometown. The coach of that program was Mark Wetmore, then a student at Rutgers University, who went on to become the legendary multiple national championship–winning coach of the University of Colorado track and cross-country teams. That's like a musically inclined third-grader taking his first piano lessons from a young Beethoven.

Running appealed to me right from the start, not only because I had a great coach but also because I liked the individual nature of running and because, well, I was really good at it. Back then I was still playing soccer, which was my first sport. One day at practice we ran a one-mile race and I finished second against a group of kids who were mostly two and three years older than I was. In that moment I realized I should probably leave the ball alone and focus on running, and thereafter I did.

At a very early point in my running life I became totally obsessed with the art and science of training, so I read every relevant piece of material I could get my hands on—magazines, training manuals, biographies and autobiographies, you name it. By age 13 I had read more about running than many college-level coaches have. At the same time, I was applying my rapidly growing pool of knowledge in training for road races, open track meets, and school events.

When I entered high school I started training even harder. I remember reading a book called *How They Train,* which detailed the workouts of the great high school runners of the '60s, like Gerry Lindgren. The one thing these guys all had in common was that they logged copious mileage, so I thought it was normal to run a lot. Before long I was running more than 100 miles a week myself.

In my junior year of high school I became an emancipated minor—my own legal guardian. I took advantage of my independence to relocate across the country to the running mecca of Eugene, Oregon. By then I was the reigning New Jersey state champion in cross-country. The following year I became the Oregon state cross-country champion and finished third in the National Championship. These results were good enough to earn me a scholarship from the University of Oregon, where I became a two-time All-American in cross-country and track and field.

I ran professionally for ten years after college. My best marathon time was 2:13, which I achieved twice. I qualified for the Olympic Trials three times and won the Columbus Marathon on two occasions. While most competitive runners would be more than satisfied with such accomplishments, I believe I was capable of much more. As a teenager I was breaking national records, but at the elite level I never even qualified for an Olympic team. The problem was that I overtrained consistently for many years and wore my body down. I was also stubbornly self-reliant, hence uncoachable, and ignored a lot of good advice from others that could have helped me perform better.

Toward the end of my career, as I began to see my mistakes clearly, I found myself thinking more and more about what I should have done differently in my training, the changes I would make in my development as a runner if I could do it all over again, and what sort of advice I would offer to today's young runners, if given the opportunity, to help them avoid repeating my mistakes and thus achieve their full potential. In short, I started thinking like a coach.

Born to Coach

I now believe that coaching is what I was really born to do. I used to think I had been born to run, but looking back I see that, as much as I loved running throughout my career, my passion for the *craft* of training was even greater. In other words, I liked coaching myself even more than I enjoyed running. My current situation as the head coach of an elite running team is thus ideal for me, because I am able to practice and develop the craft of training with several great athletes simultaneously.

The first runner I coached was Sarah Toland, who qualified for the World Cross Country Championships while I was working with her. During that period Sarah did a few of my workouts with her friend and fellow elite runner Shayne Culpepper. Impressed by Sarah's sudden improvement, Shayne later asked me to coach her. By that time I had also begun advising Steve Slattery, a steeplechaser who won a national championship with the help of some of my suggestions. When Shayne won the Olympic Trials at 5,000 meters the next year, a lot of other top runners began to take notice of what I was doing and approached me

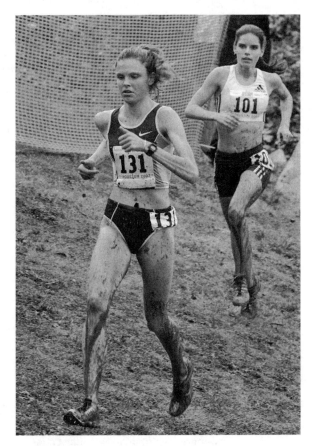

Sarah Toland © Alison Wade

to ask what I could do for them. Before I knew it I was a full-time coach.

In 2004, I created the Boulder Performance Training Group, a team of world- and national-class runners who train together under my direction. We've since moved to Eugene, Oregon, and shortened our name to the Performance Training Group. My best-known athlete is Dathan Ritzenhein, who won two National Cross Country Championships in high school and one in college and has won several big races as a professional. I am regularly forced to turn away talented runners who want to join Dathan and the others on my team, because I put so much individual time and energy into each runner that I really couldn't handle any more without sacrificing my standards.

When I started coaching, I thought that the most valuable service I would provide my runners would be to share the rich store of training knowledge I had accumulated in my head. But I have since discovered that the athletes I coach don't really need me for my knowledge of training. Ironically, they need me above all to help them *gain knowledge of themselves as runners,* because therein lies the true key to getting faster.

There are two classic mistakes that competitive runners make in their training, and both stem from an underlying failure to gather and apply self-knowledge. Mistake number one is to follow someone else's recipe for success instead of developing one's own best recipe for success based on one's individual strengths, weaknesses, needs, and goals. Mistake number two is to guide one's training too much by plans and not enough by the way one's body responds to planned training. I made both of these mistakes in my own running career. Blindly mimicking the over-the-top training habits of Gerry Lindgren and others, as I did in my teens, is a good example of mistake number one. My entire professional running career was a protracted case of mistake number two, as I refused to face the fact that my ill-fitting training patterns were destroying my body.

Without proper guidance, nearly every competitive runner commits these mistakes to some degree, as I did. Runners are always willing to work hard, but most of them have a certain lazy streak that prevents them from doing the mental work that is needed to properly customize their training and adjust it responsively day by day. Therefore my biggest job as a coach is not to show my runners the one true path to faster race times but is instead to help them discover their own, unique, ever-changing road to improvement.

The Importance of Customization

The most valuable resource that a coach can offer a competitive runner is simply another perspective. Because a coach works with many different runners, he's likely to have a better sense of the individual needs of each runner. One of the most important lessons I learned when I began coaching several runners simultaneously is how different each runner truly is. There are a great many variables, including running experience; training history; relative speed, strength, and endurance; injury patterns; recovery capacity; and others that combine to make each individual runner unique. For this reason, the ideal training approach for each runner is also unique. No two runners should train in precisely the same way.

A runner who has more natural speed than natural endurance should not train for a half-marathon the same way as a runner with more natural endurance than speed, even if the two runners have the same goal time. Similarly, a runner with one year of competitive experience should not train for a marathon the same way as a runner with twelve years of competitive experience, even if both runners share the same goal time and are the same age. These are just a couple of examples of the need for training customization that is unmet for most self-coached runners, who are never taught the importance of customizing one's training in such ways.

Fortunately for me, and for my runners, my insatiable curiosity about training methods has put me in a good position to find the right methods for each runner I work with. Many coaches are locked into a system, which is usually a modified version of the system they were taught by their own most influential coach, and they in turn apply this system to every runner they train, regardless of how each athlete responds to it. But my situation is different, because I had no single coaching mentor; instead, for the past three decades and more I have aggressively sought out and studied, absorbed, and tested every training system on earth that has produced positive results with competitive runners. As a preteen I personally met and picked the brain of the great Arthur Lydiard of New Zealand, who established the foundation of modern endurance training methods. I have since learned at the feet of dozens of other great coaches, including my former coach at the University of Oregon, Bill Dellinger, as well as Renato Canova of Italy, Steve Moneghetti of Australia, and many others. Having been exposed to such a wealth and variety of training systems, I now have a bulging bag of tricks I can draw from in developing well-customized training programs for each runner I coach.

One major advantage of trying out all kinds of different training methods is that it gives you a chance to compare them against one another. You never know if there's a better way of doing things if you keep on doing things the way you've always done them. In the process of testing various training practices, I have found that many conventional training methods simply do not work as well as alternative methods that are newer or less well known. As a result, each new runner I take on is exposed to at least one training method he or she has never used before.

The Need to Train Responsively

The key to avoiding the second common mistake related to self-knowledge that most self-coached runners make—that of not listening to their bodies—is what I call "training responsively." In my own running career I had to learn the hard way that the details of any runner's next workout should be informed 90 percent by how he or she feels after today's workout and only 10 percent by the training plan that was created before the training process actually began. So now, as a coach to other runners, I train my athletes from workout to workout instead of from training plan to training plan as I did with myself. Neither my athletes nor I know exactly what they will do in the next workout until we've assessed the state of their bodies after the most recently completed workout.

Training plans are valuable, and I do create long-term training plans for my athletes, each culminating in the individual runner's next "peak" race. But I always bear in mind that these plans necessarily make a lot of assumptions about how the runners will actually progress along the path laid out for them. For the most part, training plans represent best-case scenarios, such that, if everything goes perfectly, the runner will be able to do all of the important workouts exactly as they are planned. But nothing ever goes perfectly. Unexpected periods of fatigue crop up, muscle and joint pains emerge, and illnesses occur. Sometimes, certain components of a runner's fitness develop more slowly or even faster than expected. In either case, the workout that will do the best job of keeping the runner on track toward his or her long-term goal is not always the workout I had scheduled for that day when I sat down to map out a plan several weeks earlier.

For this reason, I plan every workout in pencil (literally and figuratively) and make a final decision about the workout at the last minute. My runners often grumble about replacing planned hard workouts with lighter ones when I determine it's necessary. And I am certain that in most cases they would go ahead and do the planned workout—usually with bad consequences—if I were not around. This is just the way runners are. It is very difficult for the typical competitive runner to truly accept the idea that backing off can be beneficial for performance. This is one reason why I believe that every runner needs to have a good coach—or learn to be a good self-coach.

If You Can't Have a Coach, Be a Coach

Every coach has some kind of training system, but the better coaches do not apply their system in the same way with every runner they work with one-on-one. Instead, they create a new, unique, highly customized training plan for each runner based on that runner's specific running experience, fitness level, and ambitions. The best coaches also watch their athletes very closely to assess how they are responding to workouts and stay ready and open to making quick adjustments—usually small ones but sometimes large—to keep their athletes on track toward their goals. It's hard work, I assure you, but these efforts to gain, share, and apply knowledge of each runner do more to help runners improve than any "system" does.

Most runners, of course, do not have the luxury of working face-to-face with a good coach every day. To achieve their goal of running faster in races, self-coached runners must find a way to become their own coach—to do for themselves what good coaches do for their athletes. Specifically, they need to learn how to create their own customized training plans that fit their individual needs, and how to tweak their training wisely from workout to workout based on how their body responds to the plan. I truly believe that learning and applying these self-coaching skills will have a greater impact on your race times than any new workout you might try or any new one-size-fits-all training plan you might find in a book or magazine. The truth is that *any* solid training system will eventually *become* the perfect training system for you if you continually customize and refine it using these self-coaching skills.

I love helping runners become faster. I get such a kick out of it that a part of me wishes I could coach every competitive runner in the entire world who has an earnest desire to improve. I wrote this book as the next best alternative. There are a lot of good running books out there that teach effective workouts and present solid training systems. But a lack of effective workouts and solid training systems is not the primary obstacle to your running faster. The primary obstacle to your running faster is a lack of self-knowledge and self-observation used specifically to customize your training methods and make smart adjustments to your training as it proceeds. In short, what's holding you back is the unfulfilled need for a second perspective—a coaching perspective—that helps put your training on track and keep it on track.

The purpose of this book is to teach you the tools you need to become your own best coach so that you can train better and run faster. Learning and applying these skills will require you to put more thought into your training than you may be accustomed to, and to pay closer attention to yourself as a runner. But, ultimately, mastering the craft of self-coaching will make your running more enjoyable and fulfilling, as well as just plain better.

I will start in chapter 1 by giving you an overview of my no-system/every-system training philosophy, which my friend and the coauthor of this book, Matt Fitzgerald, has dubbed "adaptive running." The term fits, because adaptation is the essence of my training philosophy. The goal of training, as I see it, is to stimulate the precise set of physiological adaptations that are needed to achieve maximal performance in a peak race. To achieve this objective, your training plan must be adapted based on your knowledge of yourself as a runner. Your individualized training schedule must then be adapted daily based on your response to recent training and any other factors that may affect your readiness for planned training. And finally, you must adapt your training from season to season, year to year, in response to the effects of the most recently completed training cycle (i.e., a period of training culminating in a peak race), to stimulate further positive adaptations that will help you continually develop and mature as a runner.

In chapter 2, I will present the 12 most effective training methods I have found among the hundreds I have learned and tried. These 12 practices represent the foundation for creating customized training plans. Chapters 3 through 5 cover the three basic types of training in the adaptive training system: aerobic-support training, muscle training, and specific-endurance training.

In chapters 6 through 9, we will really get down to the business of adaptation, covering the topics of how to assess your needs, strengths, and weaknesses and set goals; how to plan a fully customized training cycle; how to execute your training responsively; and how to adapt your training for year-to-year improvement. Chapter 10 ties everything together to prepare you for your self-coaching journey, and chapter 11 treats the special topic of customizing the adaptive training system to the needs of youth and masters runners.

Finally, in chapter 12, I will present a selection of training plans for each of four race distances: 5K, 10K, half-marathon, and marathon. These plans will help you get started with the adaptive approach to training and the process of becoming an effective self-coach. Just choose the plan that best fits your needs and use the tools you've learned in the rest of the book to further customize it and adjust it day by day. Before long, you will achieve a higher level of mastery over your development as a runner and you will run faster than you ever have before.

Adaptive Running

1

Every elite running coach has a training philosophy. Mine is called *adaptive running*. It is based on my belief that a responsive, evolving, creative approach to training is better than an approach that is too structured and formulaic. Simply put, there is no single training formula that works perfectly for every runner. Nor is it possible to predict exactly how a runner will respond to any particular training formula. What's more, even when a certain formula works well for a runner, he or she changes as a result of using it, so the formula must also change to produce further improvement. For these reasons, a rigid, one-size-fits-all training program will never allow you to realize your full potential as a runner. It may get you started, but it will only take you so far. Adaptive running becomes the natural way to train when you recognize that training must be customized to you individually and adapted every day based on your response to recent training.

My experience in coaching and advising a pair of elite runners—who also happen to be a married couple—provides a good illustration of why an adaptive approach to running is necessary. A few years ago, Shayne Culpepper, a 5,000-meter specialist, asked me to help her qualify for the 2004 Olympics. Shayne fared so well off the program I created for her (which you can read about in chapter 4) that her husband, Alan Culpepper, also an elite runner, decided to copy parts of it. The problem was that Alan was a completely different type of runner from Shayne. Alan has muscles that contain a lot of slow-twitch fibers; he's designed for endurance more than speed. Shayne, on the other hand, has a lot more fast-twitch fibers. Speed comes naturally to her. The training program I gave Shayne was specifically designed for a 5,000-meter runner with a lot of speed. It was not designed for a marathoner who's all slow-twitch, like Alan. Consequently, when he borrowed some of Shayne's training, Alan did not get the dramatic fitness and performance boost Shayne had gotten. Instead, he quickly became fatigued and his fitness stagnated. He tried to ignore these warning signs and push through, but the situation only worsened. Eventually, he went back to his old system, having set back his seasonal development by many weeks.

The moral of this story is twofold. First, it points to the fact that no two runners are the same. If you give two runners the same training program, they will get very different results, even if they are runners of similar ability. Alan's initial mistake was to assume that what worked for Shayne would work for him. Second, my experience with Shayne and Alan Culpepper demonstrates that runners must train responsively, modifying their

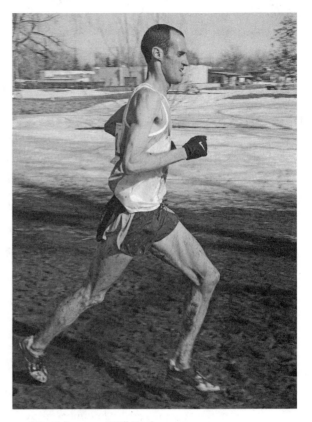

Alan Culpepper © Bill Hook

training based on how recent training has affected their bodies. Alan's biggest mistake was to persist in training Shayne's way even though it clearly wasn't working for him. Alan is actually one of the smartest self-coached runners I know, so you can be sure that if he's making these kinds of mistakes, most competitive runners are.

There are plenty of coaches and runners who understand that no two runners are the same, and that runners must adjust their training based on how they are currently feeling and performing. Yet very few coaches and runners view these realities as major considerations in the planning and execution of a training program. The typical running coach customizes the training plans he prescribes in terms of volume (miles per week), but that's about the extent of it. The rest is formulaic. Likewise, the typical competitive runner modifies her training when an injury occurs or in cases of significant fatigue, but fails to modify her training in response to subtler "surprises" (e.g., feeling unexpectedly flat on the day of a planned key workout) in the way her body responds to planned training.

The difference between my training philosophy—adaptive running—and the more typical approach to training is that I view these two lessons (first, that no two runners are the same, and second, that every runner must train responsively) of Alan Culpepper's experience as central to the planning and execution of training. I believe that there are many more factors besides the amount of running mileage a particular runner can handle that must be taken into account when creating an individually customized training plan. I also believe that planned training should be adjusted not only when major setbacks occur, but almost daily, based on a complete assessment of the runner's immediate training needs. In other words, I believe that every workout should be planned in pencil, not ink.

Imagine a spectrum that ranges from one-size-fits-all training plans at one end and made-from-scratch plans for each runner at the other end. The typical approach to training is closer to the one-size-fits-all end of the spectrum. Adaptive running is closer to the made-from-scratch end of the spectrum. Of course, there isn't a coach or runner in his right mind who believes that there is truly a single training plan that can work for every runner. Nor do I believe it makes any sense to reinvent the wheel of training for each runner. But there is a big difference between the amount of customization that the typical coach does in planning a runner's training and the amount of customization I do for my runners and recommend for self-coached runners like you.

Now imagine another spectrum that ranges from strict adherence to planned training at one end to total spontaneity at the other end. The typical competitive runner trains in fairly strict adherence to the plan, and with fairly little spontaneity. If the training plan calls for 12 quarter-mile repeats in 80 seconds apiece on Thursday, then by God, he's going to run 12 quarter-mile repeats in 80 seconds apiece on Thursday, even if he feels awful from the very first step of the workout. My approach to training encourages far more spontaneity—not arbitrary changes to the plan, but informed changes based on how the runner has responded to recent training. Naturally, there isn't a runner on earth who is completely unwilling to deviate from planned workouts. I don't advocate a make-it-up-as-you-go approach, but I do put far more emphasis on reaction and less emphasis on planning than the typical competitive runner does.

Every competitive runner trains with the objective of achieving peak-race goals. Conventional training and adaptive running are both oriented toward this objective. The difference, in my view, is that adaptive running is a more reliable way to get from point A to point B, because it entails planning the route that's best for each individual's starting place and is open to taking all kinds of helpful "detours" around unexpected obstacles along the way. In the following pages, I will give you a general overview of my adaptive running system. Subsequent chapters will provide detailed information on how to practice adaptive running in the way that works best for you.

Adaptive running is based on two rules and four principles. The purpose of the "Two Rules of Running" explained in the next section is to simplify the conceptual side of training as much as possible. These two rules are not specific to adaptive running but are truly universal: Every training system must adhere to them to be effective. In my experience, most runners fail to practice both rules as well as they should. I certainly broke them many times in my competitive days. The four principles of adaptive running discussed in the final section of this chapter represent my understanding of the best way to practice the two fundamental rules of running.

Perhaps all of this talk of rules and principles strikes you as being a bit too theoretical and not terribly practical. But the fact of the matter is that it's very important for you to get a solid mental grasp of adaptive running before you begin trying to practice it. This is because practicing adaptive running effectively requires that you take charge of your development as a runner in a way that you probably haven't before. It will oblige you to make independent decisions and solve unique problems. Simply put, it will require you—and enable you—to become your own coach. I promise you that having a solid grasp of the universal rules of running and the principles of adaptive running will help you in these situations even more than the detailed guidelines on how to practice adaptive running that you'll find in subsequent chapters.

The Two Rules of Running

Effective training can be boiled down to two simple rules. If you fully understand these rules, then adaptive running begins to make a lot of sense. And if you obey them, you will be successful as a runner. Rule one is this: Understand how the human body adapts to different types of training, and train accordingly—that is, do what works and avoid doing what doesn't work. Rule two is as follows: Learn how your *individual* body adapts to various types of training, and train accordingly—that is, do what works for *you,* and avoid doing what doesn't work for you, even if this means that you do things differently than most other runners do. Let's take a closer look at each of these rules.

Rule #1:

Understand how the human body adapts to different types of training, and train accordingly.

As I suggested above, training must be customized to the individual runner, but it doesn't need to be reinvented for every runner. Despite our many genetic and situational differences, we're all human, and our similarities really outweigh our differences. So we respond similarly to various types of training stimuli. Every runner builds greater endurance by doing longer runs. Every runner develops greater aerobic capacity by doing high-intensity intervals. No runner can run to exhaustion every day without becoming injured or overtrained. And so forth.

The sports of modern distance running, cross-country running, and track and field are a little more than a century old. Over the past eleven or twelve decades, runners and coaches have tried all kinds of training methods, with varying degrees of success. Methods that seemed to yield good results were repeated and imitated. Those that did not were usually abandoned. Contemporary training methods represent a collection of "best practices" that have survived the test of time. The general methods used by expert coaches and experienced competitive runners are proven to work well for every runner, as long as they are appropriately adapted to the individual. Making an effort to learn, understand, and base your training on our sport's "best practices" will give you the most solid possible foundation for success. It would take you more than a hundred years to find them on your own by trial and error.

Having said this much, I must add that it's also important to analyze conventional training methods with a skeptical eye, because there are some common practices that don't make a heck of a lot of sense under close scrutiny. For example, even in this enlightened age it is still common for marathon runners to use short intervals such as 400-meter repeats to "sharpen up" for a marathon in the final weeks of training. If you think about it, that's a bit like a 400-meter track specialist using 20-mile runs to "sharpen up" for a championship 400-meter race. Key sharpening workouts are most effective when they closely simulate the speed and endurance demands of your race. Thus, a *fast* 20-mile run is a better marathon sharpening workout than a set of short intervals at 3,000-meter race pace on the track. This may sound commonsensical, but many distance runners train as though the thought has never crossed their minds.

A lot of runners and coaches also make the mistake of assuming we know all we need to know about how the human body responds to training, so there's no point in trying to innovate. But I believe that effective training innovations are still possible. I spend as much time as any running coach on earth picking the brains of other top coaches and runners, studying all of the latest relevant exercise physiology literature, and making various other efforts to uncover new methods worth trying. This never-ending quest for fresh practical knowledge has led me to incorporate several unusual features into my adaptive running system that have proven beneficial for my athletes and would also be beneficial to most other runners. These methods include the use of very short, very steep, very fast hill sprints to build strength and power, and incorporating race-pace training throughout the training cycle, from the beginning of the introductory period straight through to the end of the sharpening period.

Adaptive running is the product of my exposure to a wide variety of training methods as a runner and as a student of the sport, my skeptical appraisal of even the most widely practiced methods, and my experimentation with unusual practices that seemed worth a try and proved useful. While customization, responsiveness, and evolution are major elements of adaptive running, my system also incorporates a number of standard practices that I consider the best of the best, based on my cumulative experience. Even though I train each of my runners uniquely on the level of details, on a general level there are certain characteristics that each runner's training shares with the others. These general characteristics represent the training methods that I have found to be beneficial for every runner, and therefore to be essential characteristics of any successful training program. There are 12 such general characteristics of my training method, which I will discuss in detail in chapter 2. I want you to learn and apply them all in your training, at least to start with, but you must adapt them to your individual needs, and you must not hesitate to move away from one or more of them in certain ways as you develop and learn more about what really works best for you.

Let me be clear: It's impossible to draw a clear line that marks where the universal human responses to training practices end and individual responses begin. There is plenty of disagreement even among the most experienced coaches and runners concerning which training methods truly represent the best practices that every runner should apply. Yet quite a lot is known about how the human body responds to different types of training. Learning about these cause-and-effect relationships is an indispensable shortcut to better running. Again, you will learn my take on these relationships, in the form of the 12 characteristics of adaptive running, in chapter 2.

Rule #2:

Learn how your *individual* body adapts to various types of training, and train accordingly.

In mathematics there is a concept that's called an asymptote, which is a line that moves closer and closer to another line but never meets it. When it's done right, the long-term training process is like an asymptote. The line that the training process moves toward but never reaches is "perfect training." The fact that training never meets this line symbolizes the fact that it's impossible to train perfectly. No matter how well you train, you can always look back and see something you could have done better. What's more, you're always changing as a runner—due to aging and fitness development—so you never advance beyond the need to change your training to adapt to your changing body.

While it's impossible to train perfectly, it is possible to train better and better. By learning and applying the best training practices, you can start the process pretty far along the line—much closer to perfect training than if you tried to figure out everything on your own. But you won't move any closer to perfect training unless you continually adapt your training to your individual body. The more you learn about yourself as a runner, and the more information you gather from your body's response to the training (and racing) that you do, the better you'll be able to tweak your future training to apply the right training stimulus at the right time.

You can start this custom adaptation process before you even begin your next training cycle by creating a customized training program that adapts the tried-and-true training methods to fit your specific needs. Then, once you've started the training program, you can adapt it further each day based on how your body responds to the training you've done. Once you complete the training program, you can take everything you've learned about yourself as a runner over the past weeks and apply it in creating the next training program, which will be even better customized than the one just completed. And on it goes.

Adjusting, refining, and customizing your training—in short, practicing the second rule of running—requires that you pay close attention to the results of your training and racing. Paying close attention is the only way to know when an adjustment is needed, and what sort of adjustment might be best. It's the only way to gather the knowledge about yourself as a runner that you need to refine and evolve your training so that your personal training recipe becomes ever more customized to your unique combination of strengths, weaknesses, needs, and goals.

The concept of paying close attention is simple enough, but most competitive runners are not accustomed to closely analyzing the results of their training. They prefer to do as much work as possible with their legs and as little as possible with their heads. I can understand that; it's easier just to go on automatic pilot. But your legwork will be much more effective if you make a consistent effort to use your head to practice the second rule of running and thereby make your training truly adaptive on every level.

The Four Principles of Adaptive Running

There are four ways in which your training must be adaptive. Hence there are four key principles of adaptive running. First of all, everything about your training has to be oriented toward the goal of stimulating the precise set of physiological *adaptations* that you will need to achieve your next peak-race goal. Second, the plan you create to achieve this goal must *adapt* tried-and-true training methods to fit your unique running makeup. Third, this plan must *adapt* each day based on how your body responds to planned training. And finally, your next training cycle must be *adapted* based on what you learn about yourself as a runner and your progress made in the present training cycle. Let's take a closer look at the practical applications of each of these four principles.

Adaptive Running Principle #1:

The goal of training is to stimulate the precise set of physiological adaptations that are needed to achieve maximum performance in a peak race.

Each runner has what I call a performance threshold at any given race distance—that is, a maximal average pace that he or she can sustain from the starting line to the finish line. Your objective in each cycle of training is to elevate the threshold associated with the distance of your chosen peak race. For example, if your best average marathon pace is 7:00/mile, your next training objective might be to improve your marathon threshold pace to 6:51/mile (sub-three-hour pace). To achieve this objective, you must first achieve certain specific physiological adaptations that will enable you to run faster than you have in the past.

Your training program will be most effective if you understand the nature of the adaptations you need to achieve this goal and how to train in a way that takes you from your current fitness state to the race-ready state. In other words, you need to know the physiological ingredients of better performance at your peak-race distance and the cause-effect relationships between various types of training and these ingredients. This sort of knowledge doesn't require a Ph.D. in exercise physiology. In the adaptive running system, there are only three components of running fitness: aerobic fitness, neuromuscular fitness, and specific endurance. And there are only three types of training: aerobic-support training, muscle training, and specific-endurance training. I think you can guess which type of training is used to stimulate improvement in each component of fitness.

Every race goal demands a certain level and blend of aerobic fitness, neuromuscular fitness, and specific endurance. The marathon requires a different blend of these three components than the mile does. The goal of running a three-hour marathon requires a slightly different blend than the goal of running a four-hour marathon. And the blend of aerobic fitness, neuromuscular fitness, and specific endurance that you would need to run a three-hour marathon might even be a bit different from the blend that another runner would need to achieve the same goal, based on differences in your strengths and weaknesses.

Conceptually, training to achieve your race goal is as simple as performing the right mix of aerobic training, muscle training, and specific-endurance training to develop your running fitness from its current state to the state that will enable you to sustain your target pace over the full race distance. By the time you finish reading this book, you will know how to do this with confidence.

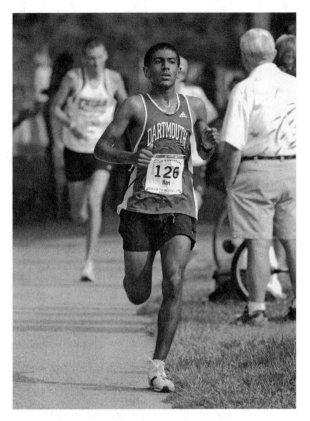

For the competitive runner, the objective of training is to adapt the body to the specific demands of racing.
© Alison Wade

Adaptive Running Principle #2:

Training programs must be adapted to the individual strengths, weaknesses, needs, and goals of each runner.

As I mentioned before, there are a number of training methods that seem to work well for all runners. Every runner should learn these methods and incorporate them into his or her training. These methods include long runs, threshold runs, and recovery (or "easy") runs. But the best ways to apply these universal principles and methods are different for each runner. In order to train optimally, you must not only understand the universals; you also must know yourself as a runner. Only then can you create a fully customized training plan that will work best for you.

When you sit down to design a training plan for yourself, begin by considering your recent training, your age and overall running experience, your goals, your injury history, your strengths and weaknesses, and other such factors that are relevant to your training. Assessing yourself in terms of these factors will allow you to create a plan that is well customized to the runner that only you are. The most important consideration is your goal. Appropriate goal-setting itself must be based on a clear-eyed assessment of your ability as a runner. I have found that most competitive runners are able to set appropriate goals if given a few simple tools to work with. When you establish a goal, you establish the set of physiological adaptations that will be needed to achieve your goal, and this, in turn, will tell you the types of peak-level training you will need to be capable of doing in the final weeks before your peak race.

The specific training path you select to get from point A (your current fitness level) to point B (your goal) will then depend on how you assess other factors, such as the running mileage that is most appropriate for you given your past training and your next goal. Other important considerations include your current place in the long-term process of development as a runner (your "running age") and whether your injury history suggests that certain measures should be taken to avoid further injuries in the future.

This assessment can be used to create a training program that's a little different from the program that any other runner might create in pursuit of the same goal. It will share many of the basic elements with other running programs, but the details will be distinct, because they will have been chosen in response to your individual assessment. In chapter 6, I will show you how to conduct your own complete running self-assessment.

Adaptive Running Principle #3:

Individualized training schedules must be adapted daily, based on the runner's response to recent training and any other factors that may affect the runner's readiness for planned training.

As I've mentioned, it's impossible to predict exactly how your body will respond to the training you have planned—even if you have done a good job of customizing your training to your strengths, weaknesses, needs, and goals. In addition, factors outside of training may also affect your body in ways that have implications for your planned training. For these reasons, a certain amount of responsive adaptation is required to stay on track toward your objective throughout the training process.

Training for a peak race is kind of like undertaking a long sailing trip. The shortest distance to your destination is a straight line, but the *fastest* way to get there will involve many zigzags. You will encounter unpredictable winds and currents on your journey. In responding to these factors, you may find yourself heading a little to the left or right of your final destination some days, but your overall progress in the right general direction will be much greater than it would be if you stubbornly insisted on heading straight toward your destination regardless of winds and currents.

Those unexpected winds and currents are like the small surprises you experience in your body's response to training as the process unfolds. Some days you feel better than expected, other days worse, and certain facets of your running fitness are sure to improve faster or slower than you thought they would. If you respond appropriately to these surprises, you will probably achieve your goal despite making many on-the-fly adjustments. If you insist on executing every workout exactly as you planned it many weeks ago, you probably won't achieve your goal.

The objective is to always try to do the most beneficial workout possible each day from the beginning of the program to the end. There are two strategies that I recommend to achieve this objective. The first is planning in pencil. By this I mean that all of the workouts you include in your training plans should be considered tentatively scheduled. These planned-in-pencil workouts represent what you anticipate being the most appropriate workouts to perform each day when you sit down to draw up a map leading to your next peak-race goal. But they are created with the understanding that you will have a much better sense of which workout is most appropriate on any given day as that day draws near. And you might not be certain about which workout is most appropriate until hours before you start warming up, or even after you've begun a workout.

Planning in pencil is different from not planning at all, of course. It is very helpful to have a concrete understanding of the training steps you will realistically have to take to develop your fitness from its current state to a race-ready state. However, it is equally important to understand the limitations of a training plan. The main limitation of training plans is that they try to predict the future based on limited data. Planning in pencil means waiting to make a final decision about the format of your next workout until you have all the data you need to make the best possible decision.

The second adaptive running strategy to ensure that you always do the most beneficial workout on any given day is responsive adjustment. Once you have gone to the trouble of creating a training plan, you should follow it. In other words, you should do the workout that is scheduled each day unless you have a specific reason to do a different workout or take a day off. Not only your decision to change your planned workout, but also your choice of a specific alternative to the planned workout, must be based on a clear assessment of your present needs. Responsive adjustment is a method of altering planned training on the basis of information provided by your own body. In practice it can range from replacing a planned hard workout with an easy run based on lingering fatigue, to adding more muscle training to your schedule based on an assessment that your neuromuscular fitness is not where it should be.

Adaptive Running Principle #4:

The runner must adapt his or her training from season to season, year to year, in response to the effects of the most recently completed training cycle, to stimulate further positive adaptations.

A training stimulus is a workout or sequence of workouts that provokes an adaptive response. A training stimulus only remains a stimulus as long as your body is still adapting to it. Once your body has fully adapted to a training stimulus, continuing to train the same way will not produce any additional fitness gains. In order to continue gaining fitness, you need to modify your training such that it will once again stimulate an adaptive response.

For this reason, you must not train exactly the same way in consecutive training cycles. No matter how much success you had in your last training program, you need to change it in sensible ways to keep improving. Put another way, you need to take advantage of the success you had in your last training cycle by creating a new training plan that demands even more from your body. I will provide comprehensive guidelines on how to adapt your training from one training cycle to the next in chapter 11.

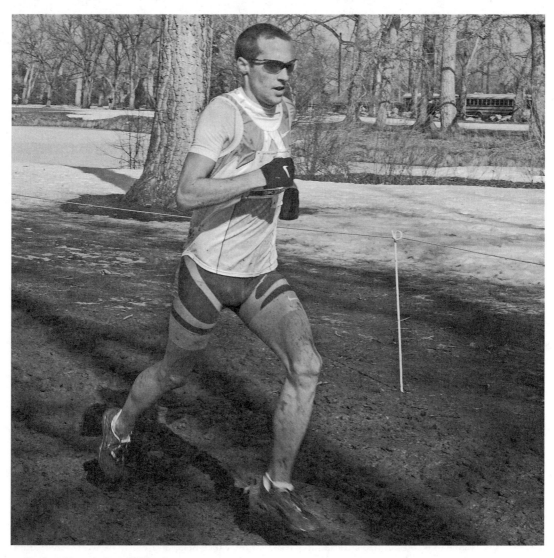

Dathan Ritzenhein © Bill Hook

Runner Profile: Dathan Ritzenhein

Dathan Ritzenhein is one of the most gifted American-born runners in history. He won back-to-back Foot Locker Cross Country National Championships in high school, claimed a World Junior Cross Country Championships bronze medal in 2001, and won the NCAA Cross Country Championships in 2004. At only 25 years of age, he has a long and bright competitive future ahead of him.

I became Dathan's coach shortly after he decided to forego his remaining NCAA eligibility and turn professional following his sophomore year at the University of Colorado. There were two main priorities I started to address when I began working with him. The first was his susceptibility to injuries. He had already suffered two stress fractures and a few other breakdowns in his short running career. Most injury-prone runners have poor muscle strength in one or more important areas, and I found this to be the case with Dathan. He had trained hard in his youth, but the biggest thing he had neglected in his training was strength. To address the problem, I had him do a lot of short, steep hill sprints. His strength improved quickly, and he's been free of major injuries for a long time now.

My second priority as Dathan's coach has been to develop his aerobic system. Aerobic development should always be an important priority for young distance runners, because it takes years of consistent training to develop the aerobic system to near-peak levels and nothing else contributes more to success in distance running than a strong aerobic system. Yet Dathan has already done a lot of running for one so young, and he has a solid aerobic foundation, so not just any workout is going to give him a stimulus for further aerobic development. The most beneficial workouts for him at this stage are challenging long runs and aggressive tempo runs. I give him as much lactate threshold training as he can handle. High-intensity intervals are administered in small doses. There will be plenty of time for more of that stuff later. The rest is filler, but it's a kind of filler that matters. High total running volume is itself a good aerobic stimulus for Dathan, as it is for any runner whose aerobic system still has potential for further development.

Dathan has responded well to this training recipe. His first race after I started working with him was a competitive international cross-country race in Ireland, which he won, beating several top African runners. More recently, he recorded personal best times at 5,000 meters and 10,000 meters on the track.

After working with Dathan for only a short period of time, I became convinced that he was really built to run fast for a couple of hours—in other words, for marathon running. One of the most important tasks in my coaching role is figuring out what type of runner each of my athletes is and using this assessment to channel him or her in the right career direction. In this case, I saw that Dathan was small and light, had predominately slow-twitch muscle fibers, and was very fatigue-resistant: a born marathon runner. I discussed these observations with him and we decided that there was no reason to wait to move him up to the marathon distance. Dathan's first marathon was a bit of a disappointment, but his second was a major breakthrough: On November 3, 2007, he took second place at the U.S. Olympic Team Trials – Men's Marathon and qualified to run in the 2008 Olympic Marathon in Beijing, China.

Adaptive Running Methods

2

Adaptive running is not about reinventing the wheel of training for each athlete. There are certain training methods that I believe to be effective for every runner. Creating a customized training plan for yourself is simply a matter of learning these methods and applying them in the way that suits you best.

Even though I train each of my runners uniquely on the level of details, on a group level there are some general characteristics that each runner's training shares with that of the others. These general characteristics represent the training methods that I have found to be beneficial for every runner, and therefore to be essential characteristics of any successful training program. There are 12 general methods that characterize my adaptive running system:

1. consistent, moderately high running volume
2. nonlinear periodization
3. progression from general training to specific training
4. three-period training cycles
5. lots of hill running
6. extreme intensity and workload modulation
7. multi-pace workouts
8. nonweekly workout cycles
9. multiple threshold paces
10. constant variation
11. one rest day per week
12. selective cross-training

Let's take a closer look at each of these methods. This chapter is meant to serve as a general introduction to the methods you will use when practicing adaptive running. You will learn all of the details you need to know to apply these methods in subsequent chapters dealing with the specifics of designing workouts and training plans.

1. Consistent, Moderately High Running Volume

General running volume—or how much you run—is the most basic parameter of training and therefore the first parameter that each runner should consider in creating a customized training plan. How many times per week should I run? How many miles per week? How much should my running volume increase from the beginning to the end of my training plan? These are the questions you need to answer before asking any others as you look ahead to your next training cycle.

The running volume that is most appropriate for you depends on your next peak-race goal, your capacity to absorb and recover from frequent runs and longer runs, and your training history. As a general rule, I recommend that runners consistently maintain a moderately high running volume relative to these individual considerations.

Some training systems are characterized by extremely high volume rather than moderately high volume. In extreme high-volume systems, runners push themselves to run as many miles each week as they possibly can. Arthur Lydiard was a persuasive proponent of extreme high-volume training. Many of America's top runners of the 1970s and early 1980s—including Frank Shorter, Bill Rodgers, and Alberto Salazar—were strongly influenced by Lydiard's philosophy and achieved great success on high-mileage training (upwards of 150 miles per week in some cases).

Other training systems are known as high-intensity systems. In these systems, training intensity, not training volume, is considered to be the true path to running success. The weekly training schedule is packed with high-speed sessions that leave runners exhausted after relatively few miles compared to the number of miles they could complete at lower intensities. High-intensity training systems are necessarily moderate-volume systems, because the more high-speed running you do each week, the less total running you can do without becoming overtrained or injured. Many great runners have achieved outstanding success on training programs that emphasized quality over quantity. American middle-distance star Alan Webb and former marathon world record holder Steve Jones of Wales are among the most noteworthy runners to have reached the top by doing a lot of high-intensity workouts and less total mileage than most of their peers. Bill Bowerman, the legendary University of Oregon coach and Nike cofounder, also used a high-intensity, moderate-volume system with his athletes.

Based on the proven effectiveness of both approaches, I like to split the difference between the extremes in volume emphasis and intensity emphasis. I believe that high running volume is indispensable for maximal aerobic development. However, high-intensity training clearly provides fitness benefits that moderate-volume training does not. Since the only way to truly maximize running mileage is to forego high-intensity training, I believe that overemphasizing mileage is a mistake. Most runners will get the best results by finding a balance between quality (intensity) and quantity (volume). So the adaptive running approach is to do as much running at various faster speeds as you can do without seriously limiting the total running volume you can absorb, and to do as much total running as you can do without seriously limiting the amount of high-intensity running you can absorb. Naturally, the precise formula is different for each runner, and finding it requires experimentation.

Another aspect of my philosophy on running volume is consistency. Some training systems entail large fluctuations in running volume throughout the training cycle. I prefer to keep the overall running volume fairly consistent throughout the training cycle while manipulating other variables to produce fitness gains. Obviously, when an athlete's recent training has been at a low volume it is necessary to gradually increase it to the level that is required for peak fitness. However, once a runner has attained this level, I like to have him or her stay relatively close to that level thereafter, except for brief off-season rest periods.

The rationale for consistency in running volume is, first of all, that it does no harm to maintain a relatively high volume year-round. As long as you take one or two breaks each year and reduce the overall workload of your training when appropriate, you won't wear yourself down. Secondly, having to build your running fitness from a low level to the level required for peak fitness can really bog down a training program, because volume increases must be executed gradually to avoid overtraining and injuries, and it's very risky to increase overall running mileage and high-intensity running mileage simultaneously. You'll be able to build fitness faster and peak at a higher performance level if you start each training cycle with a relatively high volume of running. And the only way to safely start a training cycle at a fairly high volume is never to allow your training volume to drop too low.

A third benefit of maintaining moderately high running mileage more or less year-round is that it reduces injury risk. Injuries tend to occur during periods of increasing running volume. If you keep your mileage relatively high, you will minimize these risky volume ramp-up periods in your training.

2. Nonlinear Periodization

Every running coach uses a variety of types of training with athletes. Each specific type of training is intended to develop a specific aspect of running fitness. In my adaptive running system, aerobic-support training develops the aerobic system, muscle training cultivates the neuromuscular aspect of running fitness (i.e., speed, strength, and power), and specific-endurance training is used to layer a race-specific fitness peak atop the foundation of aerobic and neuromuscular fitness. Most other training systems involve a similar mix of training types, although there are significant discrepancies in the details.

The term "periodization" refers to how one's training evolves from the beginning to the end of a training cycle. Periodization is considered linear when each period or phase of training is very different from the other periods in terms of the degree to which each training type is emphasized or deemphasized. Periodization is considered nonlinear when all of the training types are mixed together throughout the training cycle and changes in emphasis are less extreme. My approach to periodization is nonlinear.

Traditionally, linear periodization has been the more popular approach. And even today, a lot of coaches divide the training cycle into distinct phases and put a strong emphasis on just one type of training in each phase. By contrast, my training plans feature a more even balance of training types throughout the training cycle. My runners always work on every aspect of running fitness. The distribution of emphasis does change, but I do not reduce any training type to mere "lip-service" level, or phase it out entirely, as others do. The only exception is the final few weeks of training before a peak race, called the sharpening period, when we really zero in on race-pace training. I'll say more about the sharpening period later in the chapter.

I believe it's extremely important never to allow any single aspect of your running fitness to fall too far behind the others in your training, because they are all so deeply interdependent. The inevitable consequence of allowing, say, your neuromuscular fitness to stagnate while you work hard on your aerobic fitness and specific endurance is that lack of neuromuscular fitness will become a limiter to further development of the other two aspects of your fitness.

Some runners do not perform a weekly long run at the beginning of base training, but I like to introduce this type of training immediately and keep it there throughout the training cycle. Some runners do sprint training only during one brief phase of the training cycle, but my runners do sprints once or twice every week (on steep hills). In conventional training systems, lactate threshold training (described later in this chapter) is introduced in the middle of the training cycle. I prescribe threshold work from the very beginning and increase it steadily until the middle of the training cycle, after which time I may or may not taper it off, depending on the athlete's primary race distance. But it never goes away. The same general pattern holds for every type of training that's a part of the adaptive running system.

In addition to preventing weak links from developing, another advantage of nonlinear periodization is that it increases the adaptability of your training. When you keep all aspects of your running fitness at a fairly high level, you can take your training in any of a number of different directions fairly quickly based on what you seem to need. When you've recently neglected any specific type of training, it's always necessary to ease into doing more of it—otherwise you risk becoming overtrained or injured. So if you suddenly find that a lack of muscle training has left you with a deficit of neuromuscular fitness (you'll find out how to make such assessments in chapter 8), your only sensible course of action to correct this problem is to start doing small amounts of muscle training and gradually build neuromuscular fitness from its current low level. But if challenging muscle-training efforts have remained a regular part of your training, you can correct a neuromuscular fitness deficit much more quickly by aggressively boosting your muscle training without much risk of becoming overtrained (that is, chronically fatigued) or getting hurt.

3. Progression from General Training to Specific Training

One of the most important principles of sports performance is the principle of specificity. It refers to the fact that the body adapts very specifically to the demands placed upon it in training. Due to the principle of specificity, there is no such thing as truly all-around running fitness. The running fitness of every runner is always limited, reflecting the specific nature of the training he or she has done. For example, you might run 100 miles a week on the plains of Nebraska and consider yourself one heck of a fit runner, but when you compete in the Mt. Washington Road Race you get your butt kicked because your body is not specifically adapted to running up hills. Or you might be able to run a full marathon at a pace of eight minutes per mile, because you always train at this pace, but for the same reason, when you try to sustain seven-minute miles in a 10K race you come up short.

The most important ramification of the principle of specificity for competitive runners is that race-specific fitness requires race-pace training. Every competitive runner likes to achieve time goals in races. When you show up to a race with a particular time goal in mind, whether or not you achieve that goal depends on whether your body is able to sustain the average pace that is associated with your time goal over the entire race distance. The principle of specificity tells us that your body is most likely to have this ability if you have recently done some hard workouts that have challenged your ability to sustain your goal race pace. Doing highly race-specific workouts in your peak weeks of training will ensure that your body is specifically adapted to your particular race time goal.

The principle of specificity only goes so far, however. If you took this principle to the extreme, you would perform challenging race-specific workouts throughout the training cycle. The problem with this approach is that the body can only progressively adapt to this type of training for a few weeks before it reaches a temporary adaptive limit, or peak. Therefore it's crucial to have a very high level of non-race-specific running fitness before you start to do race-specific workouts. By taking the time to build your fitness to a high level with an emphasis on the types of training that serve as a foundation for race fitness, you can perform your race-specific workouts at a higher level and therefore race at a higher level. But if you start trying to do race-specific workouts in the first week of a training cycle, when your base fitness level is relatively low, you will not be able to perform these workouts at a high level, and when you reach your adaptive limit four to six weeks later, you will not have made much progress from your starting point.

The term I use for the type of fitness that is required for successful racing is *specific endurance,* which represents the ability to resist fatigue at race pace. As mentioned above, there are two other types of running fitness that serve as elements of the foundation for race fitness: neuromuscular fitness and aerobic fitness. Neuromuscular fitness is basically the ability of your brain's motor centers to efficiently activate large numbers of muscle fibers during running, which is required to achieve high speeds and to sustain high speeds in an energy-efficient manner. Aerobic fitness refers to the ability of the runner's body to use oxygen at a high rate during running. In crude terms, neuromuscular fitness is the capacity to run very fast for a short duration and aerobic fitness is the capacity to run slow or moderately fast for a long duration. Together, these capacities represent the two "extremes" of running fitness.

Specific endurance, or race fitness, represents a blend of neuromuscular and aerobic fitness. Generally speaking, the higher you can elevate your neuromuscular or aerobic fitness, the higher you can raise your specific endurance. Therefore, my adaptive running approach to the overall training cycle is to first build a foundation by focusing on the extremes of running fitness. Gradually, I bring these extremes together by adding a little more of an aerobic element to neuromuscular training and a little more of a neuromuscular element to aerobic training. Finally, in the last few weeks of training, I focus on true specific-endurance workouts performed at or very near the runner's goal race pace. In keeping with my nonlinear approach to periodization, specific-endurance training is always part of the mix, but it stays in the background until the sharpening period.

Traditionally, the term "sharpening period" (or "sharpening phase") has been used to denote a brief period at the end of a training cycle when distance runners add short, high-speed intervals to their training to "sharpen" for a race. In the adaptive running system, the sharpening period denotes a short period at the end of the training cycle when runners emphasize challenging race-pace workouts. To avoid confusion, I sometimes tell people that I don't "sharpen" my runners for racing at all, but that's not quite accurate.

4. Three-Period Training Cycles

As alluded to above, in adaptive running, the training cycle is divided into three periods, or phases. The training cycle starts with an introductory period, which lasts just a few weeks; it then moves into a longer fundamental period; and it culminates in a sharpening period.

The purpose of the introductory period is to establish an appropriate fitness foundation that will prepare you for the more challenging and focused training of the fundamental and sharpening periods. Priority number one is to gradually but steadily increase your running mileage toward the level you have targeted as your average weekly running mileage for the training cycle. This will enhance your body's ability to absorb the training of the fundamental and sharpening periods without injury or overtraining fatigue. Other priorities of the introductory period include establishing a foundation of neuromuscular fitness with very small doses of maximal-intensity running and beginning the long process of developing efficiency and fatigue-resistance at race pace with small doses of running in the race-pace range.

In the fundamental period, your training becomes increasingly specific. Your longest runs become more race-specific by first approaching race duration (if you're training for a long race) and then by becoming faster. Your fastest runs become more race-specific by generally moving toward race pace and by challenging you to sustain fast speeds for longer and longer durations.

The purpose of the sharpening period is to raise your running fitness to its peak level, or, put another way, to make your running fitness as race-specific as possible. Peaking is a mysterious art. For whatever reasons, it's just not easy to achieve one's highest possible level of performance on the day of a major goal race, despite all the care that goes into planning one's training to produce this result.

American runners at the top levels tend to run well early in the competitive season and fall flat toward the end of the season, when they should hit their peak. The reason, I believe, is that they start to do race-specific "sharpening" training too early in the training cycle. A runner's body can only progressively adapt to race-specific training for a few weeks until a limit—that is, a peak—is reached. Trying to prolong race-specific training beyond a few weeks is almost certain to result in a premature peak or failure to peak at all. For this reason, I begin the sharpening period of training just four to six weeks before the athlete's peak race occurs.

Merely limiting the duration of your sharpening period of training will not guarantee a successful peak, however. There are a few other tricks you can use to reliably increase the odds of peaking successfully. It's all about understanding the factors that tend to trigger a peak and those that tend to delay a peak, and applying each factor as appropriate.

One factor that tends to delay a performance peak is maintaining balance in one's training. A peak tends to occur when you push your fitness strongly in a single direction by heavily emphasizing a particular type of training. I take great pains to develop a high level of well-rounded fitness in my runners through balanced training before pushing their fitness in the direction of race-specificity in the final month of training.

Race-pace training is certainly included in the overall training mix before the final four weeks, but the amount is limited compared to other training paces. Then, in the sharpening phase, I have my runners really home in on the race-pace range to effect a quick, quantum leap in race-specific fitness. Now is no longer the time to be a well-rounded runner. You want to be as good as you can be at only one thing: running at your goal race pace over the full race distance.

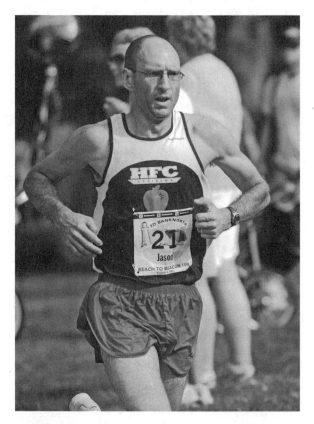

In the adaptive running system, you will maintain a consistently high level of well-rounded fitness.
© Alison Wade

If you can achieve a handful of workout performances in the sharpening period of training that are almost equivalent to your goal race performance, your attainment of that goal will be all but guaranteed (as long as you rest up adequately before the race). To achieve such workout performances, you must first of all be very close to race fitness, thanks to the training you've done up to this point; second, you must be sufficiently recovered from recent training to perform near your best; and finally, the format of the workout must be very similar to the race itself.

For example, if you're peaking for a 10K, your toughest sharpening workout might consist of 6 × 1 mile at 10K race pace with very short, 60-second active recoveries.

5. Lots of Hill Running

People who know only a little about my training system seem to know me as the coach who has his runners do a lot of hill sprints. Short hill sprints are an integral feature of my training system, and one that I use with every runner. However, this method is no more important than any of the 11 other adaptive running methods discussed in this chapter. Nor am I the only coach who uses steep hill sprints. In fact, I myself borrowed the specific approach to hill sprints that I now use from the Italian coach Renato Canova, who in turn learned about them from an American sprint coach named Bud James.

Like the other core training methods in my system, hill work is used throughout the training cycle. The amount and type of hill training varies, however. We start with very short sprints—approximately eight seconds apiece—at maximal intensity on the steepest hill we can find. The nature of this challenge is not much different from that of a set of explosive Olympic weightlifting exercises in the gym, except it is more running-specific. These short, maximal-intensity efforts against gravity offer two key benefits. First, they strengthen all of the running muscles, making the runner much less injury-prone. They also increase the power and efficiency of the stride, enabling the runner to cover more ground with each stride with less energy in race circumstances. These are significant benefits from a training method that takes very little time and is fun to do.

As the weeks go by, we gradually increase the number of sprints performed in each session. The intervals also become slightly longer (increasing to 10 seconds and finally to 12 seconds), and we may move to less-steep gradients. This process serves to make the gains in strength, power, and muscle fiber recruitment more specific to race-intensity and race-duration running.

Hill running is the only "weightlifting" my runners do. They hoist no barbells or dumbbells. They do some exercises to develop strength in their abdominal muscles and lower back, but that's it. Some other runners lift weights to build strength and prevent injuries. I believe that short hill sprints achieve the same effect. A number of the runners I've coached over the years have come to me with long injury histories, but in every such case I've been able to keep them healthy, and I attribute much of this success to hill work.

For example, for three years I coached a very talented high school runner who was also very injury-prone. Her parents brought her to me because every time she tried to take her training workload to the next level, she developed a stress fracture. When I started working with her, I had her start doing hill sprints. She quickly became noticeably stronger and her injury problems vanished. Incidentally, her best mile time dropped from 5:30 to 4:54 in one year.

In addition to hill sprints, I make frequent use of longer hill repetitions and uphill progressions. Hill repetitions are essentially speed work with an added hill component. They put less strain on the legs than traditional speed work, making them a good alternative early in the training cycle for all runners as well as for those limited by their strength. Uphill progressions are prolonged stretches of uphill running (10 minutes or more) at the end of an otherwise easy run. They are an effective way to increase the aerobic training stimulus and the strength-building stimulus of a workout without taking too much out of a runner.

6. Extreme Intensity and Workload Modulation

Intensity modulation refers to changing the pace level or levels that are targeted from workout to workout. Extreme intensity modulation means changing target pace levels more frequently and to a greater degree throughout the typical week of training than most runners do. Workload modulation refers to changing the overall challenge level of a workout from one run to the next. (Bear in mind that a high-intensity workout is not the same thing as a high-workload workout. Very fast runs can be relatively easy if they're also short, while moderate-pace runs can be quite challenging if they're long enough.) Extreme workload modulation means mixing workouts of widely varying challenge levels throughout the week.

I believe in doing two hard workouts per week, not including the weekend long run. By "hard workouts" I mean workouts involving a moderate to large dose of high-intensity running (half-marathon race pace or faster). It can be a somewhat misleading term, because the weekly long run can be the most challenging run of all for certain runners at certain times (especially toward the end of a half-marathon or marathon training program), but I've been using the term forever and I'm too old to change. I use the term "key workouts" when referring to the weekly long run *and* the twice-weekly hard workouts together.

Some elite runners try to pack in three hard workouts during the week—that is, three workouts featuring moderate to large volumes of high-intensity running. You might say that these runners train harder than my runners, who only do two. I'm not so sure. In fact, my observation has been that, over time, runners accomplish more hard training, or at least absorb more hard training, when they do two hard workouts per week instead of three. This happens because you work hardest on your best days—that is, on the days when you feel freshest and most ready. Runners are able to perform at a higher level in their hard workouts when they do just two a week because they have more opportunity to recover between them.

In simple terms, what I'm saying is that two *really* hard workouts per week are better than three *merely* hard workouts. I believe that workouts have the greatest fitness-boosting effect when they take you to a higher level of performance than you have previously achieved in the present training cycle. In order to take you to a higher performance level, the workout must be demanding in duration and intensity, but it also must occur when your body is fully up to this challenge. Having more recovery time between hard workouts enables you to perform better in each hard workout, which enhances the fitness-boosting potential of each hard workout—provided you once again give your body a chance to absorb it.

Fatigue masks fitness. When you start a workout carrying fatigue from previous workouts, you will not perform as well as you should. Consequently, the workout will have limited effect on your fitness, even if you do rest adequately afterward. Some competitive runners fear that giving themselves more opportunity to recover necessarily means that they do not train as hard. But in fact, more often than not, giving yourself adequate recovery time enables you to train harder by setting you up to perform at a higher level in your most important workouts.

In addition to limiting the number of high-intensity workouts to two per week, adaptive running also brings back the lost art of the moderate run. For many years, the motto "go hard or go home" has been an accurate representation of how most coaches approach training. Either you're doing a very hard run to stimulate fitness adaptations or you're doing a very easy recovery run to help absorb the previous hard run and prepare for the next. But a weekly schedule that entails only two hard runs makes it possible to also do one or two moderate runs (in addition to easy recovery runs) without hampering your recovery from a previous hard run or sabotaging your performance in the next.

I think it's worth taking advantage of this opportunity to do moderate runs for the simple reason that a moderate run provides a stronger training stimulus than an easy run. So if your body can effectively absorb one or two moderate runs per week in addition to two very hard runs, it just makes sense to do those moderate runs instead of the easy runs you would do according to the "go hard or go home" philosophy.

Naturally, the terms "hard," "moderate," and "easy" are relative. To give you a sense of what I mean by a moderate workout, let me supply one example. Suppose an appropriate hard workout for you at a given stage of training consists of 5 × 1K at your current 5K race pace with three-minute active recoveries, sandwiched between a two-mile warm-up and a one-mile cool-down. A typical easy recovery workout is 30 minutes of easy jogging. A moderate workout, then, might be a 15K progression run in which you run the first 10K at an easy pace and the last 5K at roughly marathon pace.

If the hard workouts tend to be especially hard in the adaptive running system, the easy workouts are often equally extreme at the other end of the workload spectrum. The single most common training error I see in competitive runners is running too hard on supposed easy days. There's no shame in running slow. Running slow allows you to run longer, and it also enables you to run harder when you want to run hard. A longer, slower

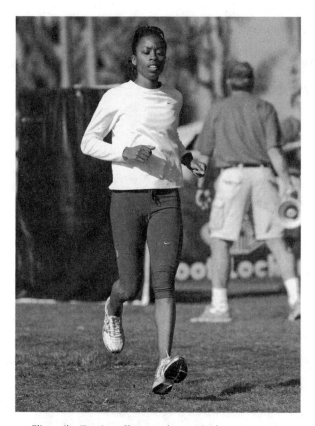

Elite miler Treniere Clement shows it's okay to run slow sometimes, even if you're very fast.
© Alison Wade

recovery run is better than a shorter, faster one, because a longer recovery run adds more volume to your training, and again, volume is the number-one determinant of running fitness.

I've also found that very slow recovery runs are less likely to leave runners feeling flat in their next hard workout, even when they are longer than the all-too-typical moderate-pace "recovery" run. Many runners fail to recover adequately from their hard workouts because they run too hard on their easy days. As a result, their performance suffers in their next hard workout. A vicious circle is formed.

Wearing a heart-rate monitor on your easy runs is a good way to keep yourself honest. By wearing a heart-rate monitor regularly in your training, you will gain accurate knowledge of the heart-rate range that is associated with a moderately easy effort. When you set out on an easy run, control your pace to keep your heart rate within that range. Your restraint will pay off the next time you're supposed to run hard.

Table 2.1 Adaptive Running Pace Levels

In running, exercise intensity is understood in terms of pace. The following table lists all of the pace targets used in adaptive running workouts and also identifies the type of training stimulus each of them provides, the type of workouts each is used in, and an example of such a workout. You will learn much more about how these target pace levels are used in adaptive running workouts in subsequent chapters.

Running Pace/Intensity	Training Type	Workouts Used In	Example Workout
Easy (a pace that feels subjectively comfortable)	Aerobic	Easy ("recovery") runs, some long runs, progression runs	Easy Run 5 miles easy
Moderate (a pace that feels comfortable with a mild aerobic strain)	Aerobic	Moderate runs, some progression runs	Progression Run 4 miles easy + 2 miles moderate
Hard (a pace that feels hard but manageable relative to distance)	Aerobic/Specific Endurance	Some progression runs	Progression Run 4 miles easy + 2 miles hard
Marathon Pace (your per-mile marathon pace in peak condition)	Aerobic/Specific Endurance	Threshold runs, marathon-pace runs	Marathon-Pace Run 2 miles easy 10 miles @ marathon pace 2 miles easy

Running Pace/ Intensity	Training Type	Workouts Used In	Example Workout
Half-Marathon Pace (either your current or goal half-marathon pace, depending on workout)	Aerobic/Specific Endurance	Threshold runs	Threshold Run 2 miles easy 2 × 15 min. @ half-marathon pace w/ 1-min. active recovery 2 miles easy
10K Pace (either your current or goal 10K pace, depending on workout)	Aerobic/Specific Endurance	Threshold runs, specific-endurance intervals, ladder intervals, hill intervals, fartlek runs	Specific-Endurance Intervals 2 miles easy 5 × 1 mile @ 10K pace w/ 400m active recoveries 2 miles easy
5K Pace (either your current or goal 5K pace, depending on workout)	Specific Endurance	Specific-endurance intervals, ladder intervals, hill intervals, fartlek runs	Hill Intervals 2 miles easy 6 × 2 min. uphill @ 5K effort w/ jog-back recoveries 2 miles easy
3K Pace (your known or estimated race pace for 3,000 meters or 2 miles	Muscle Training	Speed intervals, ladder intervals, hill intervals, fartlek runs	Fartlek Run 8 miles easy w/ 10 × 20 sec. @ 5K-3K pace
1,500m Pace (your known or estimated race pace for 1,500 meters or 1 mile)	Muscle Training	Speed intervals, ladder intervals, fartlek runs, strides	Ladder Intervals 2 miles easy 1 min., 2 min., 3 min., 2 min., 1 min., 2 min., 3 min. @ 5K–1,500m pace w/= duration active recoveries 2 miles easy
Maximal Effort	Muscle Training	Steep hill sprints	Example 5 miles easy + 6 × 8-sec. hill sprint w/ jog-back recoveries

7. Multi-Pace Workouts

Multi-pace workouts represent a training method that I use to achieve greater intensity modulation in the adaptive running system. Most traditional running workout formats focus on just a single pace, or intensity level. For example, in a standard long run, the runner holds a steady, moderate pace long enough to develop a moderate to high level of fatigue. In a standard speed workout, a runner might run 12 × 400 meters at 1,500-meter race pace.

Yes, there is also easy running in such workouts, in the form of a warm-up, a cool-down, and "active recoveries" between the hard 400-meter intervals, but this easy running only serves to facilitate the 1,500-meter-pace running, which is the one true target intensity of the workout.

Workouts featuring multiple-intensity targets are certainly not unheard-of in competitive running, but adaptive running relies on them far more heavily than most coaches do. Examples include ladder interval workouts, which may feature intervals of one minute to six minutes in duration, with the shortest intervals run at 3,000-meter race pace and the longest intervals run at 10K race pace; progression runs, in which the first segment is run at an easy (comfortable) pace and the last segment at either a steady faster pace or a gradually accelerating pace; and hybrid workouts that include threshold running at 10K or half-marathon pace and hill repetitions. What's great about such workouts is that they enable you to include more intensity variation in each week of training than you can when you force yourself to focus on a single target intensity in most workouts.

There are times in the training process when your body might benefit most from a small amount of a particular type of training, such as "speed" training at 1,500-meter to 3,000-meter pace. With multi-pace workouts, it's easy to get a small dose of speed training or another training intensity level when you need it. But if you're too reliant on traditional methods, you're faced with a choice of either devoting an entire workout to this type of training, and therefore getting more than you need, or foregoing it, and therefore not getting enough.

8. Nonweekly Workout Cycles

Another method I use to facilitate intensity modulation in training—which goes hand in hand with multi-pace workouts—is not locking myself into rigid one-week cycles. It's traditional to do one workout of any given type per week, excluding easy runs: one threshold run, one interval workout, one long run, and so forth. But there are times when, for example, you might benefit most from doing more than one threshold run per week—perhaps one-and-a-half (i.e., one long threshold run and one short one) or even two would be ideal—or less than one threshold run per week—perhaps only half a threshold workout (i.e., one short threshold run), or one every 10 days.

In the adaptive running system, it's okay to break any convention you wish to break in pursuit of getting the right amounts and proportions of training at various intensity levels. Single-pace workouts and one-week cycles are used when and only when they serve this end. When they cannot, never hesitate to use multi-pace workouts and nonweekly cycles to achieve the right mix.

9. Multiple Threshold Paces

In conventional training systems, "threshold training" refers specifically to running at a pace corresponding to one's lactate threshold (also known as the anaerobic threshold). In my adaptive running system, threshold training has a different meaning. Specifically, I deal with multiple thresholds, of which the lactate threshold is one.

The problem I have with one-dimensional threshold training is that it lacks specificity to race goals. A runner's race goal is to sustain a certain pace over a certain distance. Lactate-threshold pace—or the running pace at which the blood lactate level begins to spike—falls between 10K race pace and half-marathon race pace for most runners. Well, that's a perfectly useful training pace in some circumstances, but there's nothing magical about it. Somewhat slower and somewhat faster training paces are equally useful in other circumstances. The specific "threshold" pace that is most beneficial to a given runner at a given time depends on the race distance he or she is preparing for, the runner's goal pace, and how far along the runner is in the training process. A mistake that is made in many training systems with respect to threshold training is to overuse the lactate threshold and underutilize other alternatives.

The approach I prefer is to use at least three distinct threshold pace levels in training and to carefully sequence them to develop more and more race-specific fitness. I don't really care how much lactate my runners have in their blood at any given running pace. I care how long my runners can sustain their goal race pace and how fast a pace they can sustain over their goal race distance. The purpose of threshold training is to increase the duration a runner can sustain pace levels approaching race pace and/or to increase the pace a runner can sustain over distance.

So, what are the three threshold pace levels? The first threshold is the fastest pace the runner could sustain for 2.5 hours, or a little slower than marathon pace for my male runners. The second threshold is the fastest pace the runner could sustain for 90 minutes, which is a little faster than marathon pace for my male runners. And the third threshold is the fastest pace the runner could sustain for one hour, which is half-marathon race pace or a bit faster for my male runners.

For sub-elite runners, the three thresholds are more likely to be marathon pace or a little faster, half-marathon pace, and a little slower than 10K pace. When you practice adaptive running, you can simply run your threshold workouts at your real or estimated marathon pace (minus a few seconds per mile), half-marathon pace, and/or 10K pace (plus a few seconds per mile). There's no need for scientific precision. The advantage of the multi-pace approach to threshold training is not greater precision but greater variability, so you can do threshold workouts that are a better fit for your needs at any given time.

10. Constant Variation

Variation is intrinsic to my adaptive training system in the sense that I include several different types of workout in each week throughout the training cycle. It is also intrinsic to the progressive nature of the system. Workouts of the same type become more challenging from one week to the next to take advantage of increasing fitness and to stimulate even greater fitness gains. But I also like to include some variation for variation's sake in my training—little wrinkles in workouts that don't have any particular rationale beyond forcing the runner's body and mind to experience the unfamiliar or unexpected.

For example, on a Tuesday I might have one of my runners perform a fairly standard 10K-pace threshold run on flat roads. The next Tuesday I might have the runner cover the same distance at the same intensity level on a trail with steeply undulating hills. The next Tuesday I might move the runner back to the road and insert a 100-meter burst at 1,500-meter race pace at the end of each kilometer.

There are several benefits of such variation. Much of the fitness improvement we experience through training comes as the result of improved communication between the brain and the muscles. The brain learns to activate muscle fibers it was formerly unable to activate, discovers energy-saving ways of timing the activation of different muscles in the unfolding of the stride action, learns how to better relax muscles that don't need to be active in certain phases of the stride, and so forth. The primary factor that stimulates these sorts of learning is variation. Each time you change the way you run, your brain is forced to change the way it communicates with your muscles, and in facing this challenge your brain makes discoveries that allow you to run more efficiently and powerfully thereafter. So the more variation you can include in each week of running—within reason—the better. Pace, surfaces, gradients, duration, fatigue states, and even shoes are among the variables you can manipulate to stimulate stride refinements.

Variation also reduces injury risk. If you run at the same pace on the same surface in the same shoes all the time, the tissues of your lower extremities face a tremendous amount of repetition in the type of stress they experience. Impact forces will concentrate in the same spots to the same degree, stride after stride, workout after workout, causing damage to accumulate. Varying your training spreads the stress around more, so that no particular spot absorbs more than it can handle. The principle is similar to that which is used on some assembly lines, where workers rotate among different specific tasks to prevent carpal tunnel syndrome.

Other benefits of constant variation are less tangible. The mental exercise of dreaming up little wrinkles to incorporate into your workout each day forces your mind to engage with your training on a deeper level. You're less likely to mentally coast through your training on "autopilot"—just putting your body through each preplanned workout and moving on. The key to making adaptive running work is paying very close attention to your body's response to training, learning about yourself as a runner, and using the information you gather to steer your training in the most appropriate direction day by day. Challenging yourself to vary your training for variation's sake is a simple means of becoming more mindful of your running—of developing that internal coach's perspective that you need to excel.

11. One Rest Day per Week

Almost all of the runners I coach are at the world-class level. They are genetic lottery winners, born with the innate potential to run very fast over great distances and the ability to absorb the staggering amounts of hard training that are required to fully realize this potential. Yet none of my athletes is exempt from the need for rest. No runner has ever been capable of training hard every day of the week, every week. That's why I prescribe one day of rest per week for each of my runners (and more whenever necessary).

Rest is relative. A rest day for my elite runners might not be the same thing as a rest day for you. For them it's usually a 45-minute run at a very easy pace. For you, and for most runners, a rest day is more likely to be a day without exercise, or at most some core-strengthening exercises. The point is to set aside a day to subject your body to much less training stress than you usually do. If you normally run 12 to 15 miles a day in two workouts, at least one of which involves some high-intensity efforts, then a single, slow, 45-minute run certainly qualifies as less taxing than normal and will very likely allow you to absorb your recent training and perform well in tomorrow's training. However, runners who normally run approximately 45 minutes a day in one session will be required to run much less, engage in some gentler form of exercise, or skip exercise altogether to achieve the same benefits of absorbing recent training and preparing for the next hard workout.

Rest days play a crucial role in effective training. It's easy for competitive runners to lose perspective and think they need to run to the point of at least mild fatigue every day. But this mentality is based on a misunderstanding of how the body adapts to training stress. Simply doing a workout does not guarantee that your body will adapt to that workout. There is a difference between doing a workout and absorbing the workout. If you follow up a hard workout too soon with another hard workout, chances are your body will not have a chance to absorb—that is, change in response to—the first workout. Rest, or at least relative rest, is required to absorb a hard workout. Rest days provide this opportunity.

There is such a thing as too much rest, though. I strongly recommend that competitive runners seeking to improve their race times run six or seven times a week, even if a couple of those six or seven runs are very slow and easy. It is difficult to achieve the volume of running that is required for improvement on fewer than six runs per week. Furthermore, it's important to do some type of vigorous exercise at least six days a week simply to stay lean and maximize your overall health.

12. Selective Cross-Training

The best way to improve your running is to run. However, other types of exercise may benefit runners by improving performance, reducing injury risk, and helping them work through injuries without losing too much fitness. These days, I'm seeing more and more runners who seem to cross-train just to cross-train. I believe in a very selective approach to cross-training. I encourage my runners to do only as much cross-training as they need, when they need it.

One form of cross-training that all runners should do consistently is core-strength training. Exercises such as stomach crunches and side step-ups strengthen muscles that play key roles in stabilizing the joints during running. The more stable your knees, hips, pelvis, and spine are when you run, the less chance you have of getting injured. A little core-strength work goes a long way. I recommend doing five or six exercises two or three times each week. The most important muscles to target are those of the upper and lower back, buttocks, hips, lower abdomen, and thighs.

Alternative forms of cardiovascular exercise, such as bicycling, can be useful when running is painful or impossible due to an injury. The best way to approach alternative cardiovascular exercise is to duplicate the planned running workouts you're missing as closely as possible in whichever alternative activity you choose. For example, if you had planned to do a 10-mile progression run with the last two miles at a moderate pace, instead do a 75-minute bike ride with the last 15 minutes at a moderate intensity.

That's about all I'm going to say about cross-training in this book, because that's about all there is to it, in my approach. For more detailed guidelines on incorporating cross-training into your program, check out *Runner's World Guide to Cross-Training* by my coauthor, Matt Fitzgerald.

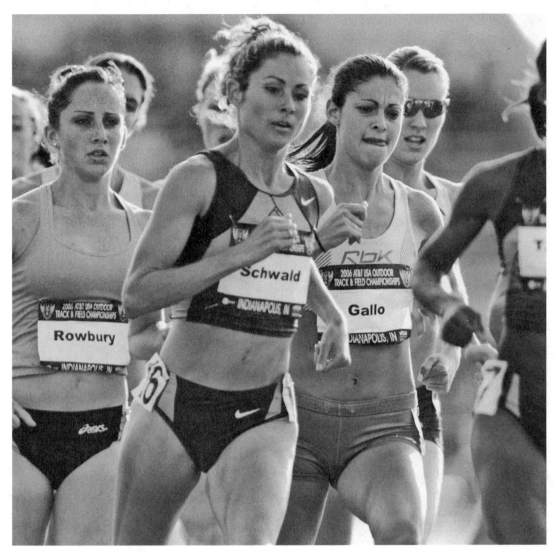

Sarah Schwald © Alison Wade

Runner Profile: Sarah Schwald

Sarah Schwald was one of the few athletes that I actively recruited. I saw her run in the 1,500 meters at the USA National Track and Field Championships in 2005. Based on close observation, I believed she was the most talented female runner at those championships, yet I also saw a lot of unrealized potential in her. She had great stride mechanics and a very elastic footstrike. I felt she would make a terrific 5,000-meter runner with proper training.

I knew that Sarah's previous coach, Peter Tegen, had heavily emphasized very high-intensity work—short intervals at 1,500-meter race pace and faster—with Sarah. To make her stronger aerobically in preparation for moving up to the 5,000, I reduced her speed training and introduced longer intervals, lots of threshold work, and more mileage. After several months on her new program, Sarah was recording workout performances that indicated she was capable of running under 15 minutes for 5,000 meters.

Unfortunately, despite her progress, Sarah left me for another coach after just one year and never did move up to the 5,000. The one mistake I made with her, I believe, was reducing her speed training a little too aggressively. Only toward the end of my time with her did I realize that she was capable of handling a fair amount of high-intensity work along with all of the aerobic stuff and, indeed, would thrive best on this mix.

My first year with any runner is mainly a learning year. I do the best I can to train the athlete optimally based on close analysis of his or her strengths and weaknesses, my knowledge of the runner's past training, and our goals. But in every case, observing the runner's response to that first year of training provides a wealth of new information that allows me to train him or her much more optimally the following year. That's why few things frustrate me more than getting only one year with a promising runner.

Expect your first year of adaptive running to be largely a learning year for you, too. Don't get me wrong: You will make plenty of progress in your first adaptive running training cycle. But in closely observing your response to this training you will learn many valuable lessons about yourself as a runner that will enable you to make substantially more progress the next time around.

Aerobic-Support Training 3

Oxygen is a big part of the sport of running. One of the signature physiological characteristics of the best distance runners is a large aerobic capacity, or the ability to consume oxygen at a very high rate while sustaining fast running speeds. And one of the primary effects of training as a distance runner is a significant increase in the ability to consume oxygen when running hard.

Why is aerobic capacity so important to running performance? Because oxygen plays a direct role in releasing energy in the muscles. The more oxygen your muscles are able to consume as you run, the more energy they can pour into moving your body forward and the faster you can run over any distance exceeding a few hundred meters.

The muscles are also able to release energy without oxygen, or anaerobically. And, in fact, anaerobic metabolism releases energy faster than aerobic metabolism does. Thus anaerobic metabolism is well suited to provide the large amounts of energy that are needed to fuel very high-intensity efforts, such as short sprints. However, anaerobic metabolism is much more wasteful than aerobic metabolism. The aerobic breakdown of a single glucose molecule yields 20 times as much energy as the anaerobic breakdown of the same glucose molecule. In addition, the aerobic system can metabolize fat, the body's most abundant energy source, whereas the anaerobic system cannot. Aerobic metabolism is therefore better suited to sustained submaximal efforts. Working muscles always release energy both aerobically and anaerobically, but the lower the intensity of exercise, the more they rely on aerobic metabolism, and the higher the intensity of exercise, the more they rely on anaerobic metabolism.

Aerobic capacity is a function of various physiological characteristics, including a large, powerful heart; high blood volume; high muscle capillary density; and high concentrations of muscle mitochondria (the intracellular sites of aerobic metabolism) and aerobic enzymes, which help oxygen break down fats and glucose to release energy. Training increases all of these factors and others related to aerobic capacity. The net result is that the runner can sustain faster and faster speeds while still relying mainly on aerobic metabolism.

Research has shown that the maximum volume of oxygen that a person can use in a given time—a figure referred to by exercise physiologists as "maximal oxygen uptake" or by the abbreviation VO_2max—accounts for roughly 70 percent of the variation in race performances among individual runners. This means that, if you are able to run a 5K one minute faster than I can, it is likely that your measured VO_2max is higher than mine by an amount that is sufficient to account for 42 seconds of that minute.

Aerobic Capacity: One Factor in the Performance Equation

As important as it is, the aerobic system is only one of two major physiological factors in the running performance equation. The neuromuscular system is the other major factor. Neuromuscular fitness, which manifests itself as stride power, stride efficiency, and fatigue resistance, affects performance as much as aerobic fitness does. Runners with very well developed neuromuscular fitness are often able to perform better than runners with a higher aerobic capacity. Studies have shown that, among trained distance runners, maximal sprint speed and broad jumping distance—two measures of neuromuscular fitness—predict long-distance racing performance as well as VO_2max does.

In the 1960s, when the concept of aerobic capacity was developed and VO_2max measurement techniques were refined, exercise scientists and running coaches got a little too excited about the whole thing and started treating oxygen consumption as the be-all and end-all of running performance. This bias led to the creation and widespread use of training practices that were designed to increase VO_2max as much as possible. The erroneous assumption underlying such aerobic-based training systems is that maximizing aerobic capacity automatically maximizes performance.

I don't believe that runners should train to maximize VO_2max or any other individual physiological variable that is related to performance. Instead, I believe that runners should train to maximize *running performance itself*, which requires that they train to develop both aerobic and neuromuscular fitness in the proper balance needed to produce *specific endurance* for their goal event (or the ability to sustain their goal race pace over the full race distance). Therefore the adaptive running approach to aerobic development is not to maximize aerobic development, possibly at the expense of neuromuscular fitness factors and/or specific endurance, but to cultivate just the right level of aerobic support to achieve race goals.

Aerobic Needs at Various Race Distances

If you were to go outside and run as far as you could in two minutes, about half your energy would come from aerobic metabolism and half from anaerobic metabolism. This makes the 800-meter run a roughly 50/50 aerobic/anaerobic event for those capable of completing this race distance in two minutes, as world-class female half-milers and upper-echelon male high school half-milers can do. You need a strong aerobic system to excel as a two-lap specialist, but you also need an equally strong anaerobic system and great speed. Every race that lasts longer than two minutes is predominantly aerobic for runners of all ability levels.

The highest rates of oxygen consumption are achieved in races of 3,000 to 5,000 meters, which test the very limits of a runner's aerobic capacity. Raw speed is still critical to success at these distances, but nothing is more important than the ability to suck down air, extract its oxygen and deliver it into the muscle mitochondria, and use the energy released there to propel forward motion. The anaerobic system still provides 20 to 30 percent of muscle energy in a 5K, however, which makes something called "lactate tolerance" another important factor in running performance at this distance. "Lactate tolerance" is a somewhat misleading term that essentially refers to the ability to resist fatigue caused by sustained anaerobic energy production, which produces chemical changes in the muscles and a level of pure pain that tend to limit performance.

When you move up to 10K, endurance factors such as running economy (or energy efficiency) and resistance to nervous system fatigue (or stride degradation—a.k.a. "falling apart") start to become more important. Aerobic capacity remains crucial, though, because the more energy you can produce aerobically, the less you have to produce anaerobically, which helps you steer around those anaerobic fatigue factors that affect 5K race performance. If 5K race performance depends on lactate *tolerance,* then you might say that 10K race performance depends more on lactate *avoidance.*

What's more, at the 10K distance, a phenomenon known as the VO_2 slow component comes into play. In maximal running efforts lasting 15 minutes or less, oxygen consumption skyrockets to a maximal or near-maximal level and then holds steady. In longer events, oxygen consumption quickly increases to an adequate submaximal level and then levels off—except it doesn't quite level off. It continues to increase slowly for the remainder of the effort as the runner fatigues. Thanks to the VO_2 slow component, you might very well find yourself breathing as hard at the end of a 10K as you do throughout a 5K.

The half-marathon is very similar to the 10K in terms of its aerobic requirements. Those endurance factors mentioned above are just slightly more important to performance at the longer distance. The marathon, finally, is a phenomenon unto itself. Roughly 95 percent of muscle energy is supplied aerobically at this distance, but the rate of oxygen consumption is well below maximal. Top competitors consume oxygen at only 85 percent of their VO_2max during a marathon, while mid-pack runners operate at closer to 75 percent of maximum. Thus, aerobic capacity is no longer quite the limiter in the marathon that it is at shorter distances.

Yet a high aerobic capacity remains essential, for three reasons. First, the faster you can run while producing roughly 75 to 85 percent of your energy aerobically, the faster you can run a marathon. Second, aerobic capacity is closely tied to endurance characteristics such as the capacity to efficiently burn fat—the most abundant muscle fuel. And third, the VO_2slow component remains in effect at this distance. You will find yourself consuming oxygen at a much higher rate in the last mile of a marathon than in the first mile, even if your pace is unchanged.

Other endurance factors that are not related to aerobic capacity are also crucial to marathon performance. These factors include running economy, resistance to running-related muscle damage, heat dissipation, and resistance to nervous-system fatigue.

So, as you can see, the aerobic requirement is different at each race distance, and it also differs somewhat between runners at any single race distance. Optimal performance at each distance requires a special balance of aerobic development and other fitness factors ranging from stride power to muscle damage resistance.

Aerobic Support

The concept of aerobic support refers to the specific foundation of aerobic system development that is best for performance at a given race distance. It's the level at which your aerobic system must be able to function to prevent oxygen delivery from limiting your performance in racing. The most practical way to conceptualize aerobic support is in terms of a specific running speed or intensity that you must ensure your body is very well adapted to in order to keep oxygen delivery from making you unable to attain your peak-race goal.

The optimal level of aerobic support for a 5K peak race is 10K pace. What this means is that you should train yourself to run a great 10K (whether or not you actually do run a 10K race) before you sharpen for a 5K peak race, because doing so is the best way to ensure that your aerobic system is not a weakness in your 5K peak race. Thus, your aerobic-support training should culminate in very challenging workouts emphasizing 10K pace running at the end of the fundamental training period.

The optimal level of aerobic support for a 10K peak race is half-marathon pace. The primary objective of your aerobic-support training, if you're training for a 10K peak race, is to cultivate a high level of half-marathon race fitness before you do your final sharpening workouts. You will achieve this objective by performing challenging workouts emphasizing half-marathon-pace running in the late fundamental period, and by training to incrementally prepare your body for these workouts throughout the whole preceding part of the training cycle.

The optimal level of aerobic support for a half-marathon peak race is also half-marathon pace. Half-marathon racing is done at or below the lactate threshold, or the pace above which anaerobic fatigue factors limit performance. As I mentioned above, aerobic capacity is paramount at this intensity level because it enables you to sustain a faster pace without submitting to anaerobic fatigue. Any pace that's slower than lactate threshold pace represents a smaller aerobic challenge, because there's no risk that anaerobic fatigue factors will come into play. That's why the optimal level of aerobic support for the half-marathon is half-marathon pace itself.

Doing too much training at race pace before the sharpening period is a sure recipe to peak too early, though, so runners training for a half-marathon peak race need to limit their half-marathon-pace training until the last several weeks of the training cycle. Their threshold workouts should feature a mix of marathon-pace, half-marathon-pace, and 10K-pace running until then.

The optimal level of aerobic support for the marathon is also half-marathon pace. Because the endurance challenge of the marathon is so severe, your goal marathon pace has to be a virtual cakewalk, aerobically. Training your aerobic system for optimal performance at the aerobically more challenging half-marathon distance is the best way to ensure that it sails through the full marathon, even if your legs don't (and they never will!).

Building Support

There are three specific jobs you must accomplish in your training to develop the level of aerobic support you need to achieve a peak-race goal. First, you must build and maintain adequate running volume, as average weekly running volume is the strongest influencer of aerobic fitness.

Second, you must develop a sufficient level of raw endurance to comfortably cover the distance of your peak race, if you do not have this level of endurance already, as is the case for most beginning runners at all distances and for runners of all experience levels at the marathon distance. Sunday long runs are the primary vehicle for the development of raw endurance in adaptive running.

Finally, you must perform workouts that are more and more challenging to your aerobic system as the training cycle unfolds. This process should culminate in the late foundation period and the sharpening period with very hard workouts emphasizing the running pace associated with the optimal level of aerobic support for your peak-race distance. Progression runs and threshold runs are the primary vehicles for the development of optimal aerobic support in adaptive running.

The Volume Question

The physiological adaptations that increase aerobic capacity are influenced by both the volume and the intensity of the running you do. The more time you spend running, the farther those adaptations will proceed. But minute for minute, higher-intensity running produces greater aerobic adaptations than lower-intensity running. So the best recipe for aerobic development is a training regimen that combines a high but manageable running volume with a fairly large volume of higher-intensity running.

That said, training volume is more foundational than training intensity with respect to aerobic development, in the sense that building up to a high volume of running with primarily moderate-intensity workouts will enable you to handle a greater amount of higher-intensity running later. For this reason, within the introductory period of the training cycle, your highest training priority should be to increase your total running mileage. By the end of this training period your running volume should be near the level at which it will remain (with some fluctuation, of course) through the remainder of the training cycle. Thus, the introductory period should last long enough to allow you to gradually build your volume to this level, without rushing the process. Beginning and less-competitive runners preparing for longer races (half-marathon and marathon) may except themselves from this rule. In such cases it's more or less necessary to build volume throughout the training cycle.

Before you start a new training cycle, you should have in mind a target average weekly training volume for the fundamental and sharpening periods. In the first week of training you should run only slightly more mileage (10 to 15 percent) than you have averaged in recent weeks, unless you're coming off a break, in which case you should use past experience and awareness of your personal limitations to determine an appropriate number of miles that you can safely handle but that will suffice to get your fitness moving in the right direction. In each subsequent week, increase your running volume by another 10 percent or so until you have reached (or at least come within 10 to 15 percent of) your volume target. Now you can move on to fundamental training.

The introductory period should not exceed six weeks, however. If you cannot build up to your target average weekly running volume level within six weeks, then your target is too high. But again, if you're a beginner or a less-competitive athlete preparing for a half-marathon or marathon, it's okay to continue building volume throughout the fundamental period.

What should your volume target be? Runners training for longer races should do more volume than those training for shorter races. One reason is that half-marathoners and marathoners need to do longer long runs to build the necessary level of endurance, but the main reason is that shorter-distance runners need to do more high-intensity running, so they are not able to put in quite as many total miles.

Table 3.1 provides guidelines that will help you select an appropriate mileage level. It presents optimal volumes for five different categories of runners at four distances. "Beginners" are runners with less than a year of consistent running under their belts. "Low-Key Competitive Runners" care about improving their race times, but are either unable or unwilling to devote a lot of time and energy to training. "Competitive" runners have at least a couple of years of hard training in their legs and are determined to improve further, but not at the cost of having to run more than six or seven times a week. "Highly Competitive" runners wish they could train like elite runners, but simply cannot. "Elite" runners know who they are. Be realistic in deciding which category you belong to. In chapter 6, which deals with the topic of self-assessment, I will offer additional guidelines to help you determine an appropriate training volume for your next training cycle.

Table 3.1 Optimal Running Volume for Five Levels of Runner at Four Race Distances					
Use this table to guide your selection of an appropriate average weekly running volume target for your next training cycle.					
	Beginner	Low-Key Competitive	Competitive	Highly Competitive	Elite
5K	20–30	25–35	40–50	50–60	90–110
10K	25–35	30–40	45–55	60–70	95–115
Half-Marathon	35–40	35–45	50–60	70–80	100–120
Marathon	40–50	50–60	60–70	80–90	110–130

If you plan to exceed 70 miles a week, you will need to run twice a day at least once a week (a practice known as "doubling"). Trying to sustain a regimen in which you average more than 10 miles *per run* places too much stress on the body, because there is no opportunity for truly easy runs, so the training workload cannot be modulated adequately.

Progression Runs, Threshold Runs, and Long Runs

Alongside overall training volume, there are three specific categories of workout that are primarily responsible for developing aerobic support at each of the four popular road-race distances. The three categories are progression runs, threshold runs, and long runs. (These workouts may also be combined, as when a 20-minute hard progression is added to the end of a long run.)

In the typical **progression run,** a short to intermediate-length segment of moderately hard (but controlled) running is added at the end of an otherwise easy run. These workouts generally serve to add a little extra aerobic challenge to a run without overly fatiguing the runner. **Threshold runs** use moderately extended running efforts at moderately high intensity levels to stimulate aerobic-system adaptations and other physiological changes that enable runners to sustain faster and faster running paces for longer and longer stretches of time. **Long runs** employ extended efforts at easy to moderately hard effort levels to build the bodily infrastructure that the aerobic system needs to work efficiently and extensively. Specifically, long runs increase muscle glycogen storage, resistance to running-related muscle damage and pain, and fat-burning efficiency.

Progression Runs

The primary purpose of progression runs is to provide a moderate stimulus for aerobic development—that is, a stronger stimulus than the typical easy recovery run but a weaker stimulus than most threshold runs. Adaptive running makes liberal use of progression runs because they represent an excellent means of squeezing a little more beneficial hard work into one's training without overtaxing the runner. Many runners rely on the aforementioned "go hard or go home mentality" in their training. Their workouts are either hard or easy—there's nothing in the middle. But I believe that a workout doesn't necessarily have to be easy if it's not hard. If you're a seven-days-a-week runner and you do two to three hard workouts per week, you probably need two to three easy days, too, but that leaves one or two days that can be moderate—and that's where progression runs come in.

Progression runs are most useful in the introductory period of training, when your fitness level is still low-to-moderate and you're not yet ready to tackle threshold workouts. Progression runs performed during this period will prepare you to benefit from tougher threshold workouts in the fundamental period. You can start with 10 minutes of moderately hard running at the end of a six- to 10-mile easy run and go from there. I like to have runners do their early progressions on an incline, or on hilly terrain, if possible, because hills build strength and it's good to build strength during the introductory period.

In the fundamental and sharpening periods, threshold workouts take on the primary responsibility of developing aerobic support. But you can continue to do one or two progression runs throughout the remainder of the training cycle, because it's all about squeezing the greatest possible benefit out of every second you spend running. If you can finish a seven-mile easy run with 10 minutes of moderately hard running without negatively affecting your performance in your designated hard workouts for a given week, why not do it?

Longer-distance runners generally should do more progression runs than shorter-distance runners should. If you're training for a 5K or a 10K, you'll want to put a heavy emphasis on training intensities exceeding those that are generally appropriate in progression runs. Half-marathon and marathon runners can make liberal use of progression runs, which emphasize running paces in the general range of race pace.

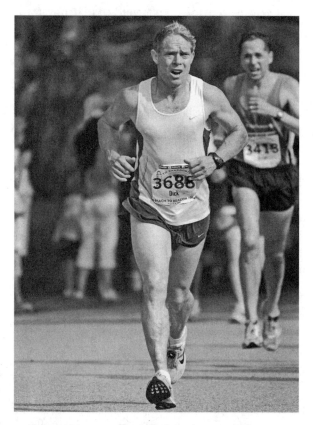

Progression runs offer a simple and manageable way to add a little extra intensity to your training.
© Alison Wade

Progressions are particularly helpful in the context of Sunday long runs in the fundamental and sharpening periods. Many runners do all of their long runs at a steady, moderate pace. Their only goal is to go the distance and build raw endurance. But for competitive runners, races are not about merely lasting to the finish line; they're about sustaining speed to the finish line. Long runs simply are not doing all that they should do if they only serve to enable you to last to the finish line. It's important to incorporate a speed challenge into some of your long runs, as well. Progression runs are a great way to do that.

I have an idiosyncratic way of prescribing intensity for progression runs. For most hard workouts, I use race-pace targets. For example, a threshold run might consist of 2×15 minutes at half-marathon pace with a 5-minute active recovery between intervals. But with progressions, I use subjective intensity guidelines: namely, "moderate" and "hard." It's important that progressions be run by feel, since their purpose is to stimulate aerobic development without exhausting the runner. It doesn't matter what pace you run in your progressions relative to your various race-pace levels. Just run at whatever pace feels "moderate" to you in workouts that call for a moderate progression, and run at whatever pace feels "hard" (yet manageable) to you in workouts that call for a hard progression. Table 3.2 presents the six essential progression runs.

Table 3.2 Progression Run Formats		
Progression Run Type	Example	Best Use
Moderate Progression Run	6 miles easy + 20 min. "moderate"	Introductory period, to prepare your body for threshold training and in later periods to squeeze a little extra hard work into your schedule
Moderate Uphill Progression Run	6 miles easy + 20 min. "moderate" (uphill, if possible)	Introductory period, to build aerobic support and strength simultaneously, or any other time you need both
Hard Progression Run	6 miles easy + 20 min. "hard"	Late fundamental period, to help coax aerobic support toward peak level
Hard Uphill Progression Run	6 miles easy + 20 min. "hard" (uphill, if possible)	Fundamental period, to build aerobic support and strength simultaneously after you've already established a foundation with moderate uphill progression runs
Long Run + Progression	12 miles easy + 30 min. "moderate"	Throughout the training cycle, to help transform race endurance into race-specific endurance
Fartlek Run + Progression	2 miles easy 4 miles: 1 min. @ 10K pace / 1 min. easy 2 miles easy 2 miles hard	Late fundamental period, as a way to incorporate two types of specific-endurance training stimulus within a longer Sunday run

Threshold Runs

Threshold training is a major part of every running coach's training system, but it is practiced differently from one system to the next. In my adaptive running system, "threshold training" refers to workouts that focus on efforts at 2.5-hour maximum pace (i.e., the fastest pace you could sustain for 2.5 hours, or a little faster than marathon race pace for most competitive runners), 90-minute maximum pace (i.e., the fastest pace you could sustain for 90 minutes, or somewhere near half-marathon race pace), and one-hour maximum pace (i.e., the fastest pace you could sustain for one hour, or somewhere between half-marathon and 10K pace). I have other workouts that focus on these pace levels—for example, long intervals at 10K pace may serve as a specific-endurance workout in the sharpening period of a 10K program—but threshold workouts always focus on one or more of these pace levels, and all of my runners do them, regardless of their race distance.

Threshold runs should be challenging, but not exhaustively so, in most cases. They are meant to provide fitness support for your toughest, most race-specific workouts, not to *be* your toughest, most race-specific workouts. You should finish your threshold workouts feeling hungry for a little more. When you incorporate well-designed threshold workouts into a nicely balanced training program, you can accomplish a hefty amount of work in these workouts and still finish them hungry.

The fitness adaptations you derive from your threshold workouts will enable you to tackle a higher workload in subsequent threshold workouts, and you should take advantage of this opportunity. You can increase the workload of your threshold workouts by making them longer (for example, advancing from 2×10 minutes at half-marathon pace to 2×15 minutes at half-marathon pace) and by making them faster (for example, by advancing from 2×15 minutes at half-marathon pace to 15 minutes at half-marathon pace plus 15 minutes accelerating from half-marathon to 10K pace). Increasing both the volume and intensity of threshold running from one workout to the next is usually not a good idea, because it increases the training stress level faster than your aerobic system can adapt.

Begin doing formal threshold runs at the start of the fundamental period. Prepare for them in the introductory period by doing a sequence of increasingly challenging progression runs. Throughout the fundamental period, increase the duration of threshold running, the pace of threshold running, or the proportion of threshold running at faster pace levels from one threshold workout to the next, except when you need or wish to reduce your workload to promote recovery or you choose to do an easier threshold run within the same week as a harder one.

Your threshold training should peak with a workout emphasizing the pace associated with the optimal level of aerobic support for your peak-race distance. The total amount of threshold running performed in this workout should represent the largest amount you can do without reaching the point of extreme fatigue. The hardest threshold workout my elite runners do is a progression of 3×15 minutes with the first effort at 2.5-hour pace, the second effort at 90-minute pace, and the third effort at one-hour pace, with 4-minute active recoveries between efforts and a long warm-up and a cool-down. A workout featuring the same basic format, but with 10- or 12-minute efforts replacing the 15-minute efforts, would be a more appropriate peak threshold workout for the average competitive runner.

An aerobic test is a special type of threshold workout that's designed specifically to assess aerobic fitness. The format I most often employ is four miles of running at half-marathon pace at the track (between a long warm-up and a cool-down). The twist is that you should wear a heart-rate monitor during this workout and control your pace not by split times but by keeping your heart rate at the level associated with half-marathon racing. Each time you repeat this workout, you should find your four-mile time improving at the same heart rate.

There are many other effective formats for threshold runs. There is no exact science to guide your selection of the most appropriate format for any given moment in your fitness development. The most important factor is the progression. If a threshold-run format moves you a step closer to the level of aerobic support you will need to achieve your peak-race goal, then it's a good workout. Table 3.3 presents four basic threshold-run formats and guidelines on their best use.

Table 3.3 Threshold-Run Formats		
Threshold-Run Format	Example	Best Use
Threshold Run (One Interval)	2 miles easy 4 miles @ half-marathon pace 2 miles easy	Do shorter versions of this workout in the early fundamental period to build aerobic support, and do longer versions in the late fundamental and sharpening periods to finish the job.

Threshold-Run Format	Example	Best Use
Threshold Run (Two Intervals)	2 miles easy 15 min. @ half-marathon pace 2 min. easy 15 min. @ 10K pace 2 miles easy	Dividing threshold running into two separate intervals is slightly easier than doing the same amount of running in one block, but it can make for a more challenging workout if you take advantage of the recovery opportunity to perform more total threshold running.
Threshold Run (Three Intervals)	2 miles easy 10 min. @ marathon pace 1 min. easy 10 min. @ half-marathon pace 1 min. easy 10 min. @ 10K pace 2 miles easy	This workout is a great way to hit all three major threshold-pace levels within a single workout.
Aerobic Test	2 miles easy 4 miles @ half-marathon heart rate 2 miles easy	This workout is a good way to measure your progress in building aerobic support.

Long Runs

The first job of the long run progression (here I'm using the word "progression" in the standard sense, which has nothing to do with progression runs) that you undertake over the course of a training cycle is to ensure that you have more than enough endurance and durability to go the distance in your peak race. This job is easily accomplished for all runners at the 5K and 10K distances. It's not too challenging for most runners at the half-marathon distance, but it certainly requires more emphasis. And at the marathon distance, it's a big job for almost every runner.

The second job of long runs is to increase the speed that runners can sustain over long distances to the level needed to achieve their race goals. If your goal is just to finish a race, as it is for many first-time marathon runners, then job 1 and job 2 of long runs are the same. In most other cases they are distinct. Different types of long runs are appropriate to each job. Workouts whose primary purpose is to increase your raw endurance, or range, should be performed at an easy pace. Workouts whose primary purpose is to boost your speed over long distances should be well within your maximal distance range.

Your first long run in the introductory period should be easy and only 10 to 15 percent longer than your longest recent run. Your longest long run should be long enough to ensure that raw endurance is not a limiter with respect to your peak-race goal. As a general rule, the longer your peak race is, the more you will need to emphasize building raw endurance with easy long runs, and the higher your initial level of raw endurance is, the more you will be able to benefit from faster long runs. Thus, inexperienced runners training to "just finish" a marathon will put the heaviest emphasis on easy long runs, while very fit runners training for a 5K peak race will put the heaviest emphasis on faster long runs.

I believe that one designated long run per week, almost every week, is the optimal frequency for all runners. Doing long runs more often will seldom enhance your endurance adaptations any further and will only get in the way of other types of training. On the other hand, doing them less often will cause your endurance to decline.

Table 3.4 presents five distinct long-run formats, an example of each, and information about the best use for each.

Table 3.4 Long-Run Formats		
Long-Run Format	Example	Best Use
Easy Long Run	14 miles @ easy pace	Introductory-period long runs for less-fit runners
Moderate Long Run	14 miles @ moderate pace	Introductory-period long runs for fitter runners; also appropriate throughout training cycle for runners preparing to "just finish" a half-marathon or marathon
Long Fartlek Run	4 miles easy 5 × 1K @ marathon pace/1K easy 4 miles easy	Provides increased intensity for long runs in late fundamental and sharpening periods
Long Progression Run	10 miles easy + 4 miles hard	Provides increased intensity for long runs in late fundamental and sharpening periods
Marathon-Pace Run	10 miles easy 6 miles @ marathon pace	Sharpening workout for marathon peak race

Aerobic-Support Training Progressions for the 5K, 10K, Half-Marathon, and Marathon

I've given you some general guidelines for using progression runs, threshold runs, and long runs to develop aerobic support for various race distances. Let's now take a slightly more detailed look at how these workouts are used to develop event-specific aerobic support across the three periods of adaptive running in preparation for peak racing of the 5K, 10K, the half-marathon, and the marathon.

The following four tables present sample training plans for each of these distances with all workouts removed except for the core aerobic-support development workouts: progression runs, threshold runs, and long runs. Note that easy runs, although a form of aerobic training that makes an important contribution to total volume, are also left out for the sake of clarity. However, weekly mileage totals are listed to show how volume contributes to aerobic-support development in the plans. Mileage levels for all four plans are appropriate for the "competitive" category of runners in table 3.1.

Also note that while the introductory, fundamental, and sharpening periods are referred to in the text accompanying each table, the training schedules are not formally divided into distinct periods, in keeping with the adaptive running characteristic of blended training periods. You can mentally distinguish the periods in an approximate manner by dividing each schedule into roughly equal thirds.

Aerobic-Support Training Progression for a 5K Peak Race

This table shows an example of the progression runs, threshold runs, and long runs that might be done in a 12-week adaptive running training plan culminating in a 5K peak race. As you can see, the overall reliance on these types of workouts is fairly light. That's because the adaptive running system makes heavy use of high-intensity fartlek runs and interval sessions for 5K training. Since those types of workouts do not count as aerobic-support training, they are not shown.

Week #	Sunday	Friday	Total Miles
1	Long Run 6 miles easy		20
2	Long Run 7 miles easy		24
3	Progression Run 8 miles, last 5 min. moderate		26
4	Progression Run 9 miles, last 10 min. moderate		30
5	Progression Run 10 miles, last 15 min. moderate		29
6	Progression Run 11 miles, last 20 min. moderate		35
7	Long Run 10 miles easy	Threshold Run 2 miles easy 3 miles @ half-marathon pace 2 miles easy	37
8	Progression Run 12 miles, last 20 min. moderate		34
9	Long Run 12 miles easy	Threshold Run 2 miles easy 2 × 2 miles @ half-marathon pace w/2-min. active recovery 2 miles easy	40
10	Long Run 12 miles easy	Threshold Run 2 miles easy 5 miles @ 10K pace w/2-min. active recovery 2 miles easy	38
11	Long Run 10 miles easy	Threshold Run 2 miles easy 3 × 2 miles @ 10K pace w/2-min. active recoveries 2 miles easy	39
12	Long Run 8 miles easy		27*

*Including peak race

Aerobic-Support Training Progression for a 10K Peak Race

This table shows an example of the progression runs, threshold runs, and long runs that might be done in a 14-week adaptive running training plan culminating in a 10K peak race. Progression runs are used not only to add intensity to Sunday long runs, as in the 5K plan above, but also during the week in the introductory period to prepare the body for threshold runs in the fundamental period. Threshold runs are relied on more heavily in this plan than in the 5K plan because the running paces targeted in threshold runs are more specific to the 10K distance.

Week #	Sunday	Friday	Total Miles
1	Long Run 6 miles easy		26
2	Long Run 7 miles easy		28
3	Progression Run 8 miles, last 20 min. moderate		30
4	Progression Run 9 miles, last 20 min. hard		33
5	Progression Run 10 miles, last 20 min. moderate	Progression Run 6 miles, last 10 min. moderate	34
6		Progression Run 7 miles, last 15 min. moderate	35
7	Progression Run 12 miles, last 30 min. moderate	Progression Run 7 miles, last 20 min. moderate	39
8	Progression Run 10 miles, last 20 min. hard	Threshold Run 2 miles easy 2 × 10 min. @ marathon/half-marathon pace w/2-min. active recovery 2 miles easy	37
9		Threshold Run 2 miles easy 2 × 15 min. @ marathon/half-marathon pace w/2-min. active recovery 2 miles easy	39
10	Progression Run 12 miles, last 20 min. moderate	Threshold Run 2 miles easy 10 min. @ marathon pace 10 min. @ half-marathon pace 10 min. @ half-marathon/10K pace 2 miles easy	41
11	Progression Run 10 miles, last 15 min. hard	Threshold Run 2 miles easy 2 x 15 min. @ half-marathon pace w/ 1-min. active recovery 2 miles easy	42

Week #	Sunday	Friday	Total Miles
12	Progression Run 12 miles, last 20 min. moderate	Aerobic Test 2 miles easy 4 miles @ half-marathon heart rate 2 miles easy	46
13	Progression Run 11 miles, last 10 min. hard	Threshold Run 2 miles easy 2 x 15 min. @ half-marathon/10K pace w/ 1-min. active recovery 2 miles easy	39
14	Long Run 10 miles easy		40*

*Including peak race

Aerobic-Support Training Progression for a Half-Marathon Peak Race

This table shows an example of the progression runs, threshold runs, and long runs that might be done in a 16-week adaptive running training plan culminating in a half-marathon peak race. There is a greater reliance on progression runs than in the shorter-distance plans. These sessions take the place of higher-intensity workouts that are emphasized at the shorter distances (but are not included in these tables, which show only aerobic-support workouts). The long runs are longer to provide adequate endurance for a race distance that is more than double the 10K distance, and the threshold workouts emphasize half-marathon pace.

Week #	Sunday	Thursday	Friday	Total Miles
1	Long Run 6 miles easy			28
2	Long Run 7 miles easy			34
3	Progression Run 8 miles, last 10 min. moderate		Progression Run 8 miles, last 10 min. moderate	40
4	Progression Run 9 miles, last 15 min. moderate	Progression Run 6 miles, last 10 min. moderate	Progression Run 8 miles, last 15 min. moderate	42

Week #	Sunday	Thursday	Friday	Total Miles
5	Progression Run 8 miles, last 15 min. moderate (uphill, if possible)		Progression Run 8 miles, last 20 min. moderate	40
6	Progression Run 9 miles, last 20 min. moderate (uphill, if possible)		Threshold Run 2 miles easy 10 min. @ half-marathon pace 5 min. easy 10 min. @ half-marathon/10K pace 2 miles easy	42
7	Progression Run 10 miles, last 20 min. hard (uphill, if possible)		Threshold Run 2 miles easy 15 min. @ half-marathon pace 5 min. easy 15 min. @ half-marathon/10K pace 2 miles easy	44
8	Progression Run 10 miles, last 30 min. moderate (uphill, if possible)		Threshold Run 2 miles easy 15 min. @ half-marathon pace 15 min. @ half-marathon/10K pace 2 miles easy	48
9	Progression Run 13 miles, last 30 min. hard (uphill, if possible)		Threshold Run 2 miles easy 15 min. @ half-marathon pace 1 min. easy 15 min. @ half-marathon/10K pace 2 miles easy	48
10	Progression Run 12 miles, last 20 min. moderate		Aerobic Test 2 miles easy 4 miles @ half-marathon heart rate 2 miles easy	43
11	Fartlek Run + Progression 2 miles easy 4 miles: 1 min. @ 10K pace/ 1 min. easy 2 miles easy 2 miles hard		Threshold Run 2 miles easy 6 miles @ half-marathon pace 2 miles easy	51

Week #	Sunday	Thursday	Friday	Total Miles
12	Progression Run 14 miles, last 20 min. moderate		Threshold Run 2 miles easy 4 miles @ marathon pace 5 min. easy 4 miles @ half-marathon pace 1 mile easy	53
13	Long Fartlek Run 4 miles easy 4 miles: 90 sec. @ half-marathon–10K pace/90 sec. easy 4 miles easy		Threshold Run 2 miles easy 4 miles @ marathon pace 4 miles @ half-marathon pace 1 mile easy	46
14	Easy Run 14 miles		Threshold Run 2 miles easy 2 × 4 miles @ half-marathon pace w/5-min. active recovery 1 mile easy	51
15	Progression Run 12 miles, last 30 min. moderate		Threshold Run 2 miles easy 15 min. @ half-marathon pace 1 min. easy 15 min. @ half-marathon/10K pace 2 miles easy	48
16	Progression Run 10 miles, last 20 min. moderate	Threshold Run 2 miles easy 4 miles @ half-marathon pace 2 miles easy		44*

*Including peak race

Aerobic-Support Training Progression for a Marathon Peak Race

This table shows an example of the progression runs, threshold runs, and long runs that might be done in a 20-week adaptive running training plan culminating in a marathon peak race. There is an even greater reliance on progression runs than in the half-marathon plan, and the long runs are longer. In the fundamental and sharpening periods there is heavy use of marathon-pace and longer fartlek runs with progressions, which serve to transform raw endurance into specific endurance for the marathon.

Week #	Sunday	Tuesday	Wednesday	Friday	Total Miles
1	Long Run 12 miles easy		Progression Run 10 miles, last 5 miles moderate	Progression Run 8 miles, last 10 min. moderate	41
2	Long Run 14 miles easy		Progression Run 12 miles, last 6 miles moderate	Progression Run 8 miles, last 10 min. moderate	46
3	Long Run 16 miles easy			Progression Run 9 miles, last 15 min. moderate	48
4	Progression Run 14 miles, last 20 min. moderate (uphill, if possible)			Progression Run 9 miles, last 15 min. moderate	53
5	Progression Run 15 miles, last 30 min. moderate (uphill, if possible)			Progression Run 2 miles easy 6 miles moderate 2 miles easy	51
6	Long Run 17 miles easy		Progression Run 10 miles, last 6 miles moderate		60
7	Marathon-Pace Run 1 mile easy 10 miles @ marathon pace + 10–20 sec./mile 1 mile easy			Threshold Run 2 miles easy 2 × 15 min. @ half-marathon pace w/2-min. active recovery 3 miles easy	55
8	Progression Run 16 miles, last 30 min. hard (uphill, if possible)		Progression Run 10 miles, last 8 miles hard	Threshold Run 2 miles easy 5 miles @ half- marathon pace 2 miles easy	59
9	Fartlek Run + Progression 6 miles easy 5 miles: 1 min. @ 10K pace/1 min. easy 1 mile easy 2 miles hard				51
10	Long Run 8 miles easy				60

Week #	Sunday	Tuesday	Wednesday	Friday	Total Miles
11	Fartlek Run + Progression 6 miles easy 5 miles: 90 sec. @ 10K pace/90 sec. easy 2 miles easy 3 miles hard			Progression Run 10 miles, last 15 min. moderate	57
12	Long Run 17 miles easy	Threshold Run 2 miles easy 6 miles @ marathon/half-marathon pace 2 miles easy			50
13	Marathon-Pace Run 2 miles easy 14 miles @ marathon pace + 10–20 sec./mile 2 miles easy			Threshold Run 3 miles easy 3 × 10 min. @ half-marathon pace w/3-min. active recoveries 3 miles easy	60
14	Long Run 20 miles easy				60
15	Marathon-Pace Run 2 miles easy 13.1 miles @ marathon goal pace 2 miles easy			Progression Run 3 miles easy 6 miles moderate 2 miles easy	50
16	Long Run 22 miles easy				60
17	Marathon-Pace Run 2 miles easy 15 miles @ marathon pace + 10 sec./mi. 3 miles easy			Progression Run 9 miles, last 6 miles accelerate from marathon pace + 20 sec./mile to marathon pace	60
18	Long Run 23 miles easy	Threshold Run 2 miles easy 2 × 15 min. @ half-marathon pace w/3-min. active recovery 2 miles easy		Marathon-Pace Run 1 mile easy 8 miles @ marathon pace 1 mile easy	62

Week #	Sunday	Tuesday	Wednesday	Friday	Total Miles
19	Marathon-Pace Run 18 miles @ marathon pace + 20–30 sec./mile			Marathon-Pace Run 1 mile easy 2 × 4 miles @ marathon pace w/5-min. active recovery 1 mile easy	51
20	Long Run 13 miles easy	Marathon-Pace Run 2 miles easy 4 miles @ marathon pace – 10 sec./mile 3 miles easy			53*

*Including peak race

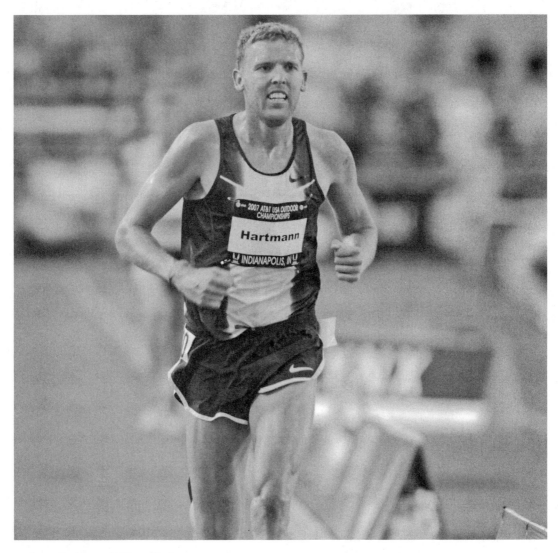

Jason Hartmann © Alison Wade

Runner Profile: Jason Hartmann

Jason Hartmann has been somewhat overshadowed by his former high school teammate, Dathan Ritzenhein, who graduated from Maryland's Rockford High School two years after Jason. But Jason is a supremely talented runner in his own right, and I am excited to be his coach.

During his college years at the University of Oregon, Jason underperformed, in part because his coach intentionally limited his training, as Jason was relatively new to running, having pursued basketball as his primary sport until his junior year of high school, and in part because of injury problems. Given this background, when Jason came to me for help in becoming an elite professional runner, I knew that we had to start by sharply increasing his mileage, to build the aerobic foundation that Dathan already had in place when he started working with me.

It takes time to build a solid aerobic foundation, so I did not race him heavily in his first year and went light on specific training, but Jason still managed to achieve some outstanding results in his first year under my guidance, including a 14th-place finish at the 2004 World Half-Marathon Championship. The terrific improvement Jason achieved with this approach underscored my conviction that younger and less-experienced runners can never go wrong by emphasizing basic aerobic training: frequent running, long runs, and lots of miles.

After Jason had a year of consistent high-volume training in his legs, I began to introduce more specific training, which has had the desired effect. He continues to get stronger, and I am confident that he will be a sub-28:00 10K runner and a 2:10 marathoner before all is said and done.

Muscle Training

4

Without a brain, you couldn't run. The act of running literally begins and ends in the brain. It begins when your brain's motor centers create electrical impulses that travel through your spinal cord and motor nerves and into your muscles, causing them to contract (or shorten). Running often ends in fatigue, which is caused mainly by a self-protective inhibition of motor impulses from the brain that occurs in response to feedback signals from the body warning of impending harm (resulting from overheating, energy depletion, loss of acid-base balance in the muscles, or another factor) if running continues. And between the beginning and the end of a run, the brain governs and regulates every process that contributes to your running, from heart rate and breathing rate to stride technique.

The physiological essence of running is two-way communication—feed-forward and feedback—between the brain and the muscles. The term "neuromuscular" is used in reference to these communications. The feed-forward part of the process happens when the brain sends electrical impulses to the muscles that cause them to contract and relax in an intricately coordinated pattern that produces the running stride. The muscles, in turn, send back to the brain a variety of signals, which provide information that helps the brain refine the running action. For example, proprioceptive nerves in the muscles and connective tissues transmit information that allows you to feel your running and react accordingly, perhaps by leaning into a steep hill. The muscles also release chemical signals that inform the brain regarding the level of acidity in the muscles, the amount of muscle damage that has accumulated, the amount of fuel remaining in the active muscles, and the temperature of the muscles.

Many of the physiological changes that lead to better running ability are neuromuscular in nature. Improvements in brain-muscle communications may increase power efficiency, running economy, and fatigue resistance.

Power

Running is not typically thought of as a power sport, but it truly is. Power is the rapid application of force. In the case of running, power has to do with the rapid application of force to the ground, which then returns this energy to the foot, propelling the body forward. The more force your foot applies to the ground, and the less time it takes to apply it, the more powerfully the ground will push your body forward.

There are several specific neuromuscular adaptations that increase stride power. The most important one is an increase in the number of muscle fibers within the working muscles that your brain can activate simultaneously. When you contract a muscle with all of your strength—for example, when showing off your biceps muscle—you may assume that all of the fibers in that muscle are active. But they are not. The average person is only able to activate roughly half of the fibers in a given muscle when contracting it with maximal effort. Training may increase the number of muscle fibers within a given muscle that you can activate simultaneously, resulting in greater maximal force and power output.

Another power-boosting neuromuscular adaptation is an increase in motor-unit firing rate. A motor unit is a bundle of muscle fibers that is fed by a single motor nerve. "Motor-unit firing rate" refers to the time that elapses between the instant your brain generates a command for a muscle to contract and the time that contraction begins. Training may shorten this span, allowing the muscles to apply force more rapidly.

Power is always movement-specific, meaning that improved power in one activity does not automatically transfer over to other activities. This is partly due to the fact that a portion of power gains is accounted for by improved coordination, and different activities require different coordination patterns. So the best way to improve running power is by running and by doing other exercises that are very similar to running, such as single-leg jumping drills.

The best distance runners are able to produce more power in the stride action than average runners can. Yet the best distance runners are not able to generate as much stride power as the best sprinters. The reason is that power is just about the only thing that is needed for performance in short sprints, whereas power is just one of several requirements for success in distance running. As we saw in the previous chapter, distance runners also need a high aerobic capacity. To some degree, however, aerobic capacity and power are mutually exclusive, because maximal-power efforts derive almost all of their energy from anaerobic metabolism. Thus, if you spend too much time training to increase your maximal stride power, you will enhance the anaerobic characteristics of your running muscles at the expense of their aerobic characteristics and your improvements in aerobic capacity will be limited.

Distance runners must also be economical, meaning that they must use energy very efficiently. Some of the physiological changes that increase maximal power reduce efficiency, starting with muscle growth. Top sprinters tend to have large muscles and relatively high body weights. But body weight and running economy are inversely related. The more you weigh, the more energy is required to run at any given speed. Therefore distance runners don't really want to improve their raw power so much as they want to increase what I call their *power efficiency*. In other words, they want to increase the amount of stride power they can generate at the highest level of energy expenditure (or oxygen consumption) that they can sustain for the entire distance of a race.

Every race exceeding 200 meters is run at a submaximal power-output level. In a 1,500-meter race you might sustain an average of 60 percent of maximal stride power from start to finish. In a marathon the figure will be closer to 40 percent. There are two power-related ways to improve your race time at any distance. First, you can increase your maximal stride power in a way that does not diminish the average percentage of maximal stride power output that you can sustain throughout the race. For example, suppose that, by incorporating a small amount of maximal-power training into an adaptive running program targeting a marathon peak race, you increase your maximal sprint speed from 7.5 meters per second to 7.8 meters per second—a 4-percent improvement. Because your program is well balanced, your power gains do not come at the expense of aerobic capacity or running economy, so the percentage of maximal power that you can sustain in a marathon remains unchanged. As a result, your marathon time will probably improve by roughly 4 percent. Thus, if your previous best marathon time was 3:00:00, your next marathon might be completed in 2:52:48.

A second power-related way to boost your running performance is to increase the average percentage of your maximal power output that you can sustain throughout a race. You will achieve this effect by following a training program that increases your aerobic capacity and running economy through high volume and challenging aerobic workouts and just enough training at very high intensities to prevent a decline in maximal stride power.

By following a well-balanced training regimen that features a little more than the minimal amount of high-intensity training, including some maximal-power work, you can achieve both of the above-described benefits simultaneously: improved maximal stride power and an increase in the average power level you can sustain in races.

Economy

The term "running economy" refers to the energy cost of running at a given speed. Reducing the energy cost of running at your goal race pace will help you sustain that pace all the way to the finish line. There are three interrelated neuromuscular changes that enhance running economy.

The most fundamental change is improved stride technique. The frequent and varied practice of the running stride that comes with a good training program leads to all kinds of adjustments in stride technique, most of them fairly subtle, which reduce the energy cost of running. For example, proper training may reduce a tendency to overstride—that is, to reach the leg out in front of the body and touch the foot to the ground heel first instead of making ground contact flat-footed with the foot directly underneath the body. Including technique drills as a regular component of your training will provide an additional stimulus for technique improvement.

A second neuromuscular adaptation that improves stride economy is a stiffening of the stride. The human body acts as a sort of spring during running. When your foot hits the ground, impact forces are sent from your body into the ground and are immediately returned from the ground into your body, providing forward propulsion. A stiff spring is more efficient than a loose spring because it delivers and receives impact force very quickly, so that little of this energy is lost through dissipation. In the same way, a runner who makes ground contact with a stiffer leg and body is likely to be more economical than a "looser" runner. In this case, stiffness comes from a tensing of the muscles in the moment preceding footstrike, resulting in a faster energy return from the ground and less energy loss through dissipation. Stiffness also enhances the stability of the knee, hip, and pelvis, minimizing the amount of impact energy that is lost through unwanted lateral movement at these joints while the foot is in contact with the ground.

Approximately half of the energy that is used to propel a runner forward is not supplied by muscle metabolism but is instead "free energy" supplied by impact forces. When the foot hits the ground, various muscles and tendons stretch beyond their natural length, capturing energy from impact forces. As these tissues return to their normal length, they release the energy, providing an impulse for forward movement. A runner with a stiffer stride may get slightly more than 50 percent of the energy required to run at a given speed from the ground, while a runner with a looser stride may get less. Proper training increases stride stiffness and the contribution of "free" elastic energy to forward movement, and hence improves running economy. The specific types of training that increase stride stiffness most are short hill sprints, power drills such as skipping, and short, fast intervals.

Training also reduces the amount of wasteful muscular "co-contraction" that occurs during running. Co-contraction is the tensing of muscles opposing the working muscles at various points in the stride action. For example, during the swing phase of the stride, when the thigh is moving forward, the hip flexors (the muscles that connect the thigh to the torso on the front of the body) are the primary working muscles. The gluteal muscles of the buttocks are directly opposed to the hip flexors. Their job at this point of the stride is to relax and stretch. Any tension in the gluteal muscles will create resistance requiring the hip flexors to work harder to pull the thigh forward. A certain amount of co-contraction is necessary at most times to stabilize joints and guide the direction of movements, but less experienced and less fit runners exhibit excessive co-contraction that does nothing but waste energy.

Training causes a natural reduction in unnecessary co-contraction that enhances running economy. You don't have to make any special efforts in your training to reduce wasteful co-contraction in your stride. It will diminish automatically as a result of your maintaining a high or relatively high volume and including plenty of variation in your program.

Fatigue Resistance

A neuromuscular phenomenon known as "motor-unit cycling" is very important in relation to running endurance. This phenomenon involves the rotating activation of individual motor units in the working muscles over the course of a prolonged running effort. During running, only 20 to 30 percent of the motor units in your working muscles are active simultaneously. But it's not the same 20 to 30 percent of motor units that are active throughout a run. On the contrary, most of the motor units in the working muscles contribute to the running effort at various times over the course of a run, but none are active all the time. Instead, they take turns: While some are active, others rest, awaiting their next turn. This cycling of motor units allows you to run much farther than you could if any of the motor units in your working muscles were forced to remain constantly active.

Training produces refinements in motor-unit cycling that increase endurance. Different cycling patterns are used at different intensities of running, so the biggest improvements in endurance will come at the running intensities you emphasize most in your training.

In every runner, there are many motor units in the running muscles that the brain seldom or never uses. These least-preferred motor units are those that contain the largest numbers of fast-twitch muscle fibers, which are normally called upon in two circumstances: when a maximal-intensity effort is demanded, and when a large number of the more-preferred slow-twitch muscle fibers are already tired from previous activity.

Increasing the total number of motor units that your brain is able to activate during running gives a boost to motor-unit cycling by creating a larger pool of motor units that can be called upon, resulting in more rest time for each motor unit in the pool. The two types of training that are most effective in expanding this pool are maximum-intensity efforts such as hill sprints and very long runs.

Muscle Training Defined

I use the term "muscle training" to denote training practices whose primary purpose is to stimulate neuromuscular adaptations that enhance running performance. Strictly speaking, *every* type of workout constitutes muscle training in the sense that every type of workout has some effect on the neuromuscular system. But as a practical matter, I prefer to limit the definition of muscle training to workouts and drills that increase stride power and fatigue resistance at faster speeds. There are three general groups of training methods that fit this definition: hill sprints and hill repetitions; speed intervals; and strides and drills.

The characteristic that unites all of these training methods is that they entail very high-intensity, largely anaerobic efforts. They call for the nervous system to activate very large numbers of motor units, to fire these motor units quickly, to contract the muscles with great force, and to resist fatigue at maximal and near-maximal intensity levels. They test the limits of the neuromuscular system's capacity to generate and sustain running-specific speed and power and thereby push back these limits. By engaging in regular, progressive muscle training, you will improve your brain-muscle communications in ways that increase your power efficiency, running economy, and fatigue resistance.

Muscle training represents half of the foundation that supports specific endurance, or the physiological capacity to run the full distance of a race at your goal pace. The other half of this foundation is, of course, aerobic support, which was discussed in the previous chapter. To achieve a higher level of specific endurance, you must first build a higher level of aerobic support and neuromuscular fitness. Broadly speaking, aerobic-support training and muscle training move toward specific endurance from opposite ends of the spectrum of running fitness. If the most foundational sort of aerobic-support workout is a long run at a slow pace (or better yet, a whole week of long runs at a slow pace), then the most foundational sort of muscle-training effort is an all-out sprint lasting only a few seconds.

The general progression pattern of muscle training is the same for all runners, regardless of their peak-race distance. The first priority is to increase maximal running-specific strength and stride power. Next, power and strength are transformed into speed. Finally, speed is gradually extended into specific endurance. A small amount of work is done to maintain power and strength as the training focus turns toward speed and then specific endurance, and to maintain speed as the training focus turns toward specific endurance.

Short hill sprints are the primary means of first increasing and then maintaining specific strength and stride power. Hill repetitions help to build a "fitness bridge" between strength and speed. The primary tool for speed development is speed intervals, or short intervals run at 5K pace and faster. Strides, which consist of very short (about 100-meter) intervals, usually at 1,500-meter pace, are essentially a form of speed interval used in warm-ups and cool-downs. Drills are also used in warm-ups and serve to develop and maintain power efficiency.

Let's now take a closer look at each of these three groups of muscle-training methods. Then I will show you how these methods are used in the adaptive running system to develop race-specific neuromuscular fitness for the 5K, 10K, half-marathon, and marathon.

Hill Sprints and Hill Repetitions

If you have never done a steep hill sprint before, you should not leap into a set of 10 steep hill sprints the very first time you try them, especially if you are over age 30. These efforts place a tremendous amount of stress on the muscles and connective tissues. Thus, the beginner is at some risk of suffering a muscle or tendon strain or another such acute injury when performing steep hill sprints. Once your legs have adapted to the stress that steep hill sprints impose, this workout actually protects against injury. But you must proceed with caution until you get over the hump of those early adaptations.

The whole point of steep hill sprints is to demand a truly maximal-power effort. For this reason, they should be very short. Your first session, performed after completion of an easy run, should consist of just one or two 8-second sprints on a steep gradient of approximately 6 to 8 percent. If you don't know what a 6- to 8-percent gradient looks or feels like, get on a treadmill and adjust the incline to 6 percent. After you've had the experience of running on this gradient, you can find a hill that matches it.

Your first session will stimulate physiological adaptations that serve to better protect your muscles and connective tissues from damage in your next session. Known to exercise scientists as the "repeated bout effect," these adaptations occur very quickly. If you do your first steep hill sprint workout on a Monday, you will be ready to do another session by Thursday—and you will almost certainly experience less muscle soreness after this second session.

Thanks to the repeated bout effect, you can increase your steep hill sprint training fairly rapidly and thereby develop stride power quickly. First, increase the number of 8-second sprints you perform by one or two per session per week. Once you're doing 8 to 10 sprints, you may move to 10-second sprints and a slightly steeper hill. After a few more weeks, you may advance to 12-second sprints on a 10-percent gradient, if you feel the need to further increase your stride power. Always allow yourself the opportunity to recover fully between individual sprints within a session. In other words, rest long enough so that you are able to cover just as much distance in the next sprint as you did in the previous one. Simply walking back down the hill you just ran up should do the trick, but if you need more time, take it.

Most runners will achieve as much strength and power improvement as they can get by doing 10 to 12 hill sprints of 10 to 12 seconds each, twice a week. Once you have reached this level and have stopped gaining strength and power, you can cut back to one set of 6 to 10 hill sprints per week. This level of maximal power training will suffice to maintain your gains through the remainder of the training cycle.

Hill repetitions—as opposed to short hill sprints—may be used in the later introductory period and early fundamental period to build a fitness bridge between strength and speed. There are two types of runner who benefit most from hill repetitions. For very "fast-twitch" runners who specialize in shorter races and tend to peak quickly when they start doing intensive speed work on the track, hill repetitions represent a way to delay the introduction of intensive speed work and to further elevate the runner's fitness level before intensive speed training begins. Hill repetitions are also beneficial for injury-prone runners, and especially those who tend to get injured when running fast. Running at high intensities uphill involves less impact force and less tissue strain than running at the same intensity on level ground. In addition, hills add a strength-boosting element to running at high intensity that reduces injury susceptibility.

Four to six relatively short hill interval sessions will suffice even for those runners who need them the most. It's not the type of training that you should belabor, because it's really meant to be transitional. Here's a very basic example of a sensible four-week hill interval progression:

Week 1: 6 × 200 meters
Week 2: 6 × 300 meters
Week 3: 6 × 400 meters
Week 4: 5 × 600 meters

These sessions may be performed after an easy run or a long warm-up or after a threshold run. Run your hill repetitions on a somewhat shallower gradient than your steep hill sprints (4 to 6 percent). Do shorter hill repetitions (200–300 meters) at roughly 1,500-meter effort and longer ones (400–600 meters) at roughly 3K effort. Time each repetition to make sure you aren't slowing down in the later intervals. As with steep hill sprints, allow yourself to recover fully between hill repetitions. Jogging very slowly back down the hill should do the trick.

After you've completed four to six hill repetition sessions in the later introductory period and/or early fundamental period, you should be ready to take on some challenging interval workouts at the track. That said, you don't necessarily have to wait until you've completed all the hill repetition training you plan to do before you start running intervals on the track or level ground. But don't go full-bore with your speed work until you've had a chance to benefit from your hill repetition workouts, and avoid overtaxing yourself by trying to jam too much anaerobic training into your schedule.

There is seldom a need to return to hill repetitions later in the training cycle, once you've turned your attention to running fast on level ground. However, you can and should go back if you feel that track intervals are breaking your body down, or if you find that you lack sufficient specific strength.

Speed Intervals

Speed intervals are short or relatively short intervals run faster than 5K pace. Intervals run *at* 5K pace are sometimes used as speed training and sometimes used as specific-endurance training, depending on the context, and sometimes they serve both purposes simultaneously. For example, I am more inclined to consider the shorter 5K-pace intervals that a 5K runner does early in the training cycle as speed training (i.e., muscle training) and the longer 5K-pace efforts with short recoveries that the same runner does later in the training cycle as specific-endurance training. The bottom line is that the line separating speed training and specific-endurance training is fuzzy for runners training for shorter events.

In many training systems, road racers, even including marathoners, perform "speed workouts" consisting of large numbers of short, fast intervals and concentrate these workouts in a specific phase that focuses on speed development training. The adaptive running system is very different in this regard. Conventional speed workouts are used sparingly in my system, and there is no concentrated phase of speed development. Short, fast intervals are sprinkled throughout my programs, and while they are somewhat concentrated in the early foundation period, you'll never see my runners doing 400-meter repeats at 1,500-meter pace every Tuesday for six straight weeks in this stage of training, as plenty of other runners do.

In my system, the purpose of speed intervals is to provide neuromuscular fitness support for specific endurance. To do this optimally, speed intervals must be performed regularly throughout the training cycle, but they are never needed in large amounts. There are three patterns of progression in speed-interval training that combine to provide optimal neuromuscular fitness support for specific endurance. First, there should be a general movement from shorter and faster intervals toward longer and slower (but still fast) intervals. Second, speed training should become more and more integrated with specific-endurance training. And third, the overall emphasis on speed training should decrease to a minimal level in the sharpening period, especially for longer-distance runners.

I like to introduce speed intervals very early in the training cycle in the form of fartlek intervals. These usually consist of 20- to 60-second efforts at 1,500-meter to 10K pace. The precise duration and pace do not matter particularly. Progression is achieved by increasing the duration of the efforts (from 20 seconds in the first session to 25 in the next, and so forth) and by increasing the number of efforts. Fartlek intervals occur within the context of easy aerobic runs, since aerobic base building is also a major priority of the introductory training period. For the sake of developing aerobic fitness, the total duration of these runs should also increase from week to week. Fartlek runs are best performed in a pleasant environment, such as quiet roads or smooth trails, to forestall any tendency to get too "serious" about them.

In the fundamental period, it's time to get serious about interval training. Again, speed intervals in the 5K to 1,500-meter pace range must be used in a way that serves to progressively develop specific endurance, and from this perspective, there is no sense in going to the track and running huge numbers of 200-meter to 400-meter speed repetitions at 1,500-meter pace. You don't need to maximize your efficiency and fatigue resistance at 1,500-meter pace to run your best half-marathon, or even your best 5K. What you need instead is to progressively blend what speed you have with the fatigue resistance you will need to sustain your goal pace over the full race distance. This requires a deeper integration of running at paces exceeding race pace into the rest of your training than is seen in training systems where an intensive block of speed training precedes a completely separate block of more specific interval training.

There are two general types of workouts in which 5K- to 1,500-meter-pace running is used in the fundamental and sharpening periods: repetition intervals and ladder workouts.

Repetition intervals are intervals of a uniform distance and intensity: for example, 10 × 400 meters at 3K (or 2-mile) race pace with 2-minute jogging recoveries. They are useful in systematically transforming speed into specific endurance. You start with a workout comprising shorter, faster intervals at the beginning of the fundamental period and gradually increase the length and reduce the pace of the intervals throughout the fundamental period. If you're training for a 5K, your intervals will become no slower than 5K pace, which, again, lies at the boundary between muscle training and specific-endurance training. If you're training for a 10K, half-marathon, or marathon, your repetition intervals will increase further in length and slow down to 10K pace, and will thus no longer constitute muscle training, by my definition.

You can sustain a maintenance level of speed training in your schedule by doing a smaller number of speed intervals (or even just one longer speed interval) as an add-on at the end of a workout emphasizing slower running. For example, a good specific-endurance workout for the 10K is 4 × 2K at 10K pace with 1-minute jogging recoveries plus 1 × 1K at maximal effort. This workout is most effective during the sharpening period, when training at or very near 10K goal pace is the highest priority and only a very small amount of faster muscle training is needed to provide neuromuscular support.

For half-marathon and marathon runners, speed training in the fundamental and sharpening periods may take the form of add-on repetition intervals almost exclusively. For example, you might run a set of 4 to 8 × 300 meters at 3K pace after a threshold run every other week. As the duration of your threshold workouts increases, the number of add-on repetition intervals will decrease.

Ladder workouts are workouts featuring a series of intervals arranged in order of ascending distance and decreasing pace, or descending distance and increasing pace, or both. Ladder workouts represent an effective way to integrate speed training with specific-endurance training. One of my preferred ladder workouts consists of time-based intervals arranged as follows: 6 minutes, 5 minutes, 4 minutes, 3 minutes, 2 minutes, and 1 minute, with 1 minute of "active recovery" jogging at a very slow pace between intervals. The first interval is run at roughly 10K pace. Each subsequent interval is run at a pace slightly faster than that of the last, with the final 1-minute interval run at roughly 1,500-meter pace. This is a good workout for the early part of the fundamental period, when your specific-endurance training need not yet be terribly specific.

Shorter, faster ladder workouts may be used to provide a periodic dose of speed training throughout the fundamental period. For example, run intervals of 1 minute, 2 minutes, 3 minutes, 2 minutes, 1 minute, 2 minutes, and 3 minutes, at 1,500-meter to 5K pace, with active recoveries of equal duration following each interval. Run the shortest intervals fastest and the longest intervals slowest.

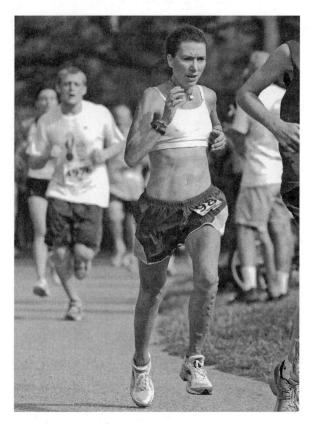

A little speed training goes a long way in the adaptive running system. © Alison Wade

It's a good idea to run a workout of this sort to establish a speed performance baseline at the beginning of the fundamental period. Thanks to the hill work and fartlek intervals you've done in the introductory period, you should be able to perform fairly well in such a workout at this time. Your objective is to sustain the level of speed performance you exhibit in this baseline workout throughout the remainder of the training cycle, even as your training becomes more and more race-specific. Repeating the ladder once every few weeks should suffice to ensure that your speed is holding steady, and it will give your speed the necessary boost if it has slipped.

Below are three basic speed-interval workout formats and guidelines for their best use.

Table 4.1 Speed-Interval Workout Formats

Speed-Interval Workout Format	Example	Best Use
Repetition Intervals	6 × 800m @ 5K pace	Done once a week with intervals becoming progressively slower and longer, these workouts transform speed into specific endurance.
Ladder Intervals	6 min., 5 min., 4 min., 3 min., 2 min., 1 min. @ 10K–1,500m pace w/1-min. jog recoveries	Ladders with longer intervals such as this one nicely integrate speed and specific endurance in the early fundamental period; ladders with shorter intervals provide a good periodic dose of speed stimulus throughout the fundamental and sharpening periods.
Add-On Intervals	20 min. threshold run @ half-marathon pace + 4 × 300m @ 3K pace	These intervals provide a small, regular dose of speed training and may be virtually all the speed training that is needed for half-marathon and marathon runners in the fundamental and sharpening periods.

Strides and Drills

Strides and drills serve somewhat different muscle-training functions, but I lump them together here because I tend to lump them together in the training of my runners. Specifically, I have my runners perform strides and drills as part of their warm-up on high-intensity running days (typically Tuesdays and Fridays). First they do some easy jogging. Then they complete a set of drills and strides. The main workout comes next, and lastly they do a cool-down consisting of more easy jogging.

The reason I place strides and drills in this context is that they do an excellent job of preparing the body for fast running—especially after you prepare your body for strides and drills with an easy jog. Strides and drills elevate muscle temperature and release appropriate hormones to a level that is conducive to efficient, fast running. They also increase muscle and connective tissue elasticity and active range of motion in the hips.

Finally, drills and strides "prime" the nervous system for fast running. Have you ever noticed that when you run a set of intervals at the track, your first and second intervals are never your best? That's because the nervous system must be primed for optimal performance.

In addition to serving as good warm-up tools, drills and strides provide general neuromuscular-fitness benefits. Strides develop neuromuscular coordination and efficiency at high speed. Drills enhance dynamic flexibility, stride power, stride stiffness, and efficiency. And one drill in particular, sideways skipping, reduces injury risk by strengthening the important stabilizing muscles at the inside and outside of the hips.

Do a set of drills and strides following the jogging portion of your warm-up in any workout involving running at 10K pace or faster. Start with one set (that is, do each drill and one stride one time) and progress to two or three sets. Following are descriptions of how to do strides and my recommended drills.

Slow Skipping

Drive your right knee upward hard. Allow the upward momentum generated by this movement to lift your left foot off the ground and take a small hop-step forward with that foot. Lower your right foot to the ground one step ahead of the left and immediately drive the left knee upward, taking a hop-step forward with the right foot. Continue skipping forward for 30 meters, leaping as high as you can with each skip. This drill increases stride power and stride stiffness.

High Knees

Run forward at a fast tempo but a slow rate of forward progress and with exaggerated knee lift. Concentrate on keeping your spine straight as you lift your thighs to a 90-degree angle to the ground. Stay up on your toes when you make ground contact. Continue moving forward for 30 meters. This drill increases dynamic flexibility in the hips and stride stiffness at the ankles.

Butt Kicks

Run at a slow rate of forward progress while trying to keep your thighs locked in line with your torso and touching the heel of your foot to your butt with each stride. Continue for 30 meters. This drill strengthens the hamstrings and increases dynamic flexibility in the knee.

Sideways Jumping Jacks

Do a regular jumping jack, but when you push off the ground, push a little harder with the right foot so you travel about a foot to the left in midair. Continue skipping sideways to the left for 30 meters, then reverse your direction and skip back to where you started. This drill strengthens the hip abductors (on the outsides of the thighs) and the hip adductors (on the insides of the thighs), enhancing the stability of the hips, pelvis, and lower spine during running and thus increasing efficiency and reducing injury risk.

Strides

Run 100 meters at approximately 1,500-meter race pace. Concentrate on keeping your stride compact, relaxed, and powerful. As mentioned above, strides help to develop neuromuscular coordination and efficiency at high speed.

Muscle-Training Progressions for the 5K, 10K, Half-Marathon, and Marathon

The optimal muscle-training progression is similar for all of the standard road-race distances from 5K to the marathon. It is a type of training that all road racers need to do regularly but that none needs to do in large amounts. In this section, I'll present 11 tables designed to illustrate the specific type of muscle training that is appropriate at various points throughout the training cycle for runners preparing for peak races at the four popular road-race distances. The tables also suggest how muscle training should be integrated into the overall training schedule.

Within each table, muscle-training elements appear in **boldface.** These elements are also described in greater detail than workouts representing other types of training, which are not our concern in this context.

Early Introductory Period—5K to Marathon

All runners, regardless of their race-distance focus, should approach muscle training similarly in the introductory period, so these first two tables—presenting representative weekly schedules for the early and late introductory period—apply to runners preparing for a peak race at any distance from 5K to the marathon.

Sunday	Long Run
Monday	Easy Run + **Hill Sprints** **(2 × 8 sec. on 8% grade)**
Tuesday	Threshold Run
Wednesday	Easy Run + Moderate Progression
Thursday	Easy Run + **Hill Sprints** **(2 × 8 sec. on 8% grade)**
Friday	Fartlek Intervals 2-mile warm-up 2 miles moderate **w/6 × 30 sec. @ 5K pace** 2-mile cool-down
Saturday	Off

Late Introductory Period—5K to Marathon

The introductory period is intended to be relatively short (three to six weeks), so there isn't a tremendous amount of progression that can occur. Developing maximal specific strength and stride power is a major muscle-training emphasis throughout the introductory period. Since this type of training must be introduced gently, however, there is significant progression in the volume of hill sprinting performed between the beginning and the end of this period.

Sunday	Long Run + Moderate Progression
Monday	Easy Run + **Hill Sprints** **(8 × 8 sec. on 8% grade)**
Tuesday	Threshold Run

Wednesday	Easy Run + Moderate Progression
Thursday	Easy Run + **Hill Sprints** (**8 × 8 sec. on 8% grade**)
Friday	Fartlek Intervals 2-mile warm-up 4 miles moderate **w/10 × 45 sec. @ 5K pace** 2-mile cool-down
Saturday	Off

Early Fundamental Period—5K

Because 5K runners race at a pace that is close to the pace of speed intervals, they need to take their own approach to the speed/specific-endurance training progression in the fundamental period. They should start with a focus on 3K-pace running to build immediate speed support for their 5K goal pace, with an optional lighter emphasis on hill repetitions, to help transform strength into speed, as illustrated in Friday's workout below. Hill sprint training may be reduced from two sessions per week to one session.

Sunday	Long Run + Moderate Progression
Monday	Easy Run + **Hill Sprints** (**10 × 10 sec. on 8% grade**)
Tuesday	Threshold Run
Wednesday	Easy Run + Moderate Progression
Thursday	Easy Run + **Strides**
Friday	**Speed Intervals + Hill Repetitions** **Strides and Drills** **4 × 400m hills @ 3,000m pace w/2-min. jog recoveries** **4 × 200m hills @ 1,500m pace w/2-min. jog recoveries**
Saturday	Off

Early Fundamental Period—10K and Half-Marathon

Runners preparing for 10K and half-marathon races should do essentially the same sorts of muscle training in the foundation period, as the same level of neuromuscular fitness support is needed for success at both distances. (For the typical runner, 10K pace is only 7 or 8 percent faster than half-marathon pace.) In this example of early fundamental-period training below, Friday's workout provides a spectrum of training stimuli ranging from specific endurance (the 6-minute interval is run at 10K pace) to extended speed (the final, 1-minute interval is run at 1,500-meter pace after only a minute's recovery).

Sunday	Long Run + Moderate Progression
Monday	Easy Run + **Hill Sprints** **(10 × 10 sec. on 8% grade)**
Tuesday	Threshold Run
Wednesday	Easy Run + Moderate Progression
Thursday	Easy Run + **Strides**
Friday	Ladder Intervals **Strides and Drills** 2 × (6 min., 5 min., 4 min., **3 min., 2 min., 1 min.**)
Saturday	Off

Early Fundamental Period—Marathon

Marathon runners don't need to mess around much with speeds exceeding 5K pace. Monday's hill sprints suffice to maintain specific strength and stride power, while Thursday's and Friday's strides administer a very small but adequate dose of running at 1,500-meter pace. Friday's repetition-intervals workout qualifies as both speed and specific-endurance training for the marathon runner at this stage.

Sunday	Long Run + Hard Progression
Monday	Easy Run + **Hill Sprints** **(10 × 10 sec. on 8% grade)**
Tuesday	Threshold Run
Wednesday	Easy Run + Moderate Progression
Thursday	Easy Run + **Strides**
Friday	**Specific-Endurance/Speed Intervals** **Strides and Drills** **6 × 800m @ 5K pace w/90-sec. jog recoveries**
Saturday	Off

Late Fundamental Period—5K

By the end of the fundamental period, hard threshold running and moderately hard specific-endurance workouts at goal pace have become the top training priorities for the 5K runner. But speed remains an important secondary priority, as evidenced by the set of 300-meter intervals at 1,500-meter pace following Tuesday's threshold workout.

Sunday	Moderate Run + Threshold Run
Monday	Easy Run + **Hill Sprints** **(10 × 10 sec. on 8% grade)**
Tuesday	Threshold Run + **Speed Intervals** **(4 × 300m @ 1,500m pace)**
Wednesday	Easy Run + Moderate Progression
Thursday	Easy Run + **Strides**
Friday	Specific-Endurance Intervals (at 5K goal pace) **Strides and Drills**
Saturday	Off

Late Fundamental Period—10K and Half-Marathon

Everything is just slightly different in this example of late-fundamental-period training for 10K and half-marathon runners as compared to the 5K example above. The longer-distance runners do a different sort of long run on Sunday, most likely a somewhat different threshold run on Tuesday, and a slower, longer specific-endurance intervals session on Friday. And as for muscle training, the short speed session following the threshold run on Tuesday also features intervals that are a little slower and a little longer than those done by the 5K runner.

Sunday	Long Run + Hard Progression
Monday	Easy Run + **Hill Sprints** **(10 × 10 sec. on 8% grade)**
Tuesday	Threshold Run + **Speed Intervals** **(3 × 400m @ 3K pace)**
Wednesday	Easy Run + Moderate Progression
Thursday	Easy Run + **Strides**
Friday	Specific-Endurance Intervals (at 10K goal pace) **Strides and Drills** 8 × 1K @ 10K pace
Saturday	Off

Late Fundamental Period—Marathon

Speed was a relatively low priority for the marathon runner in the early fundamental period and it remains so in the late fundamental period. While all marathon runners should be open to tackling a solid stint of speed training as necessary at this point in the training cycle, this more typical example includes just one add-on speed interval at 5K to 3K pace in Friday's specific-endurance workout.

Sunday	Easy/Moderate/Hard Progression
Monday	Easy Run + **Hill Sprints** **(10× 10 sec. on 8% grade)**
Tuesday	Threshold Progression 15 min. @ marathon pace 10–15 min. @ half-marathon pace 10–15 min. @ 10K pace
Wednesday	Easy Run + Moderate Progression
Thursday	Easy Run + **Strides**
Friday	Specific-Endurance Intervals + **Add-On Speed Interval** **Strides and Drills** 4 × 2K @ 10K pace + **1K @ 5K–3K pace**
Saturday	Off

Sharpening Period—5K

In the short (four- to six-week) sharpening period as much running as possible should be concentrated close to goal race pace. However, the ability to run efficiently at slightly faster speeds is crucial to provide neuromuscular-fitness support for peak 5K performance, so a block of 1,500-meter-pace running is included in Tuesday's specific-endurance workout.

Sunday	Moderate Run + Threshold Run
Monday	Easy Run + **Hill Sprints** **(10 × 10 sec. on 8% grade)**
Tuesday	Specific-Endurance + Speed Intervals **Strides and Drills** 4 × 1K @ 5K pace **4 × 400m @ 1,500m pace w/3-min. jog recoveries**
Wednesday	Easy Run + Moderate Progression
Thursday	Easy Run + **Strides**
Friday	Specific-Endurance Intervals (at 5K goal pace) **Strides and Drills**
Saturday	Off

Sharpening Period—10K and Half-Marathon

Power efficiency and fatigue resistance at goal pace are by far the most important fitness concerns in the sharpening period for 10K and half-marathon runners. The ability to resist anaerobic fatigue factors associated with faster speeds is a small aspect of neuromuscular support for 10K and half-marathon race performance. Therefore, the sample week below includes a lot of running at half-marathon and 10K pace and only strides and a single 1K add-on interval to provide a speed stimulus.

Sunday	Easy/Moderate/Hard Progression
Monday	Easy Run + **Hill Sprints** **(10 × 10 sec. on 8% grade)**
Tuesday	Threshold Run 10–15 min. @ marathon pace 10–15 min. @ half-marathon pace 10–15 min. @ half-marathon/10K pace
Wednesday	Easy Run + Moderate Progression
Thursday	Easy Run + **Strides**
Friday	Specific-Endurance Intervals + **Add-On Speed Interval** **Strides and Drills** 4 × 2K @ 10K pace + **1K @ 5K–3K pace**
Saturday	Off

Sharpening Period—Marathon

For marathon runners, efforts at 5K to 1,500-meter pace can more or less disappear in the sharpening period, as they do in this example, save for Thursday's strides.

Sunday	Marathon-Pace Run
Monday	Easy Run + **Hill Sprints** **(10 × 10 sec. on 8% grade)**
Tuesday	Specific-Endurance Intervals 4 × 3K @ half-marathon pace
Wednesday	Easy Run + Moderate Progression
Thursday	Easy Run + **Strides**
Friday	Cruise Intervals 2 × 4 miles @ marathon pace
Saturday	Off

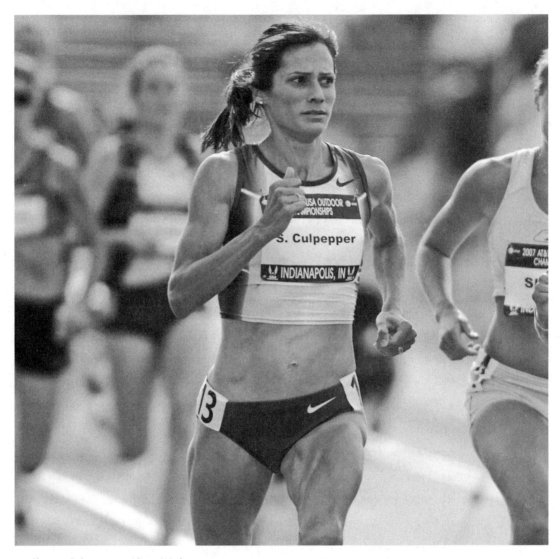

Shayne Culpepper © Alison Wade

Runner Profile: Shayne Culpepper

A few years ago, one of America's top female distance runners, Shayne Culpepper, took a year off to have a baby. When she returned to running, she decided to find a new coach. Shayne wanted more than just to return to the level she'd been at before her pregnancy— she wanted to become even better. And she was smart enough to know she would have to change her training in one or more ways to reach the next level.

Shayne allowed me to look over four years of her training logs and offer feedback. I came away from my analysis of her training logs with some definite ideas about what she needed to do differently in her training. She liked my ideas and decided to work with me.

Shayne had eight years of consistent training under her belt, which was great. But I noticed that too much of her training was at the extremes. She had done a lot of moderate aerobic training and a lot of short, fast stuff on the track, but not much in between. As a result, she was aerobically strong and had excellent speed, but she lacked the specific endurance she needed to succeed at her primary event distance of 5,000 meters. She could run 15 miles at six-minutes-per-mile pace, but struggled to run five miles at 5:30 pace.

Her goal was to qualify for the 2004 Athens Olympics at 5,000 meters. The qualifying standard was 15:08, and her best time then was 15:23. So she needed to make a fairly big step forward. To complicate matters, she didn't want to go to Europe to qualify for the Olympic Trials in the summer track meets, so we knew she had to qualify in May in the United States. We only had five months, so there was really no time to create a long, periodized program.

Fortunately, because she was 30 years old and had trained consistently for so long, Shayne did not require a lot of base work, which allowed us to get specific very quickly. After six weeks of introductory training, we went right to specific endurance. I brought in the stuff she was missing from day one: longer intervals (repeats ranging from 800 meters to 2K) and intensive threshold training.

We did two hard workouts each week. On one of her hard days I would give her 5K-specific stuff or a mix 5K-specific and 1,500-meter-specific stuff, alternating between the two formats from week to week. (The 1,500 was Shayne's secondary event.) On the other hard day she did threshold work. I had her run at half-marathon pace one week (for example, 2 times 15 minutes or 30 minutes straight at half-marathon pace) and at 10K pace the next week (2K's or 3K's at 10K race pace).

Shayne responded very well to this program. She won an IAAF World Indoor Track and Field Championships bronze medal after only two and a half months on the adaptive running system. In late May she blew away the Olympic qualifying standard for 5,000 meters, running 15:01. In July she won the Olympic Trials 5,000 meters, and she was able to live her dream of competing in the Athens Olympics.

Specific-Endurance Training

5

In the sport of distance running, it is not speed that limits us. It's endurance. The average competitive runner is capable of running world-record 5,000-meter pace. Sure, you might not be able to sustain that pace for more than 100 meters or so, but in the strictest sense it is not a lack of speed that prevents you from breaking the world record for 5,000 meters but a lack of fatigue resistance at the required speed.

When we think of endurance, we generally think of the capacity to cover vast distances and to keep moving for long spans of time. But in fact, endurance is the ability to resist fatigue at *any* level of exercise intensity, including maximal intensity. Both the 100-meter sprint and the 200-meter sprint are maximal-intensity running events, yet some sprinters who excel at 100 meters do not fare as well at 200 meters because they are unable to sustain maximal intensity as well as other sprinters who excel at both distances.

In short, every runner needs to have some measure of endurance—even those whose races last only 10 or 20 seconds. To be more precise, every runner needs to develop a level of endurance that enables him or her to sustain the highest possible percentage of maximal running speed over the full race distance. Thus, endurance is specific to each race distance. At the (male) world-class level, a 100-meter sprint specialist must be able to sustain 100 percent of his maximum sprint speed for 10 seconds. A 5,000-meter runner must be able to sustain nearly 60 percent of his maximum running speed for 13 minutes. And a marathon runner must be able to sustain roughly 40 percent of his maximum sprint speed for two hours and 10 minutes.

I use the term "specific endurance" to denote the type of endurance that is needed to maximize performance at a particular race distance. It is the ability to resist fatigue at your goal pace for a particular race distance long enough to reach the finish line without slowing down.

To achieve your race time goals, you must first attain the requisite level of specific endurance in your training. Whether or not you actually achieve your race goal times depends on other factors, as well, such as good pacing, mental toughness, and favorable weather and course conditions. But without the requisite level of specific endurance, none of these other factors matter. Achieving specific endurance for a peak race requires that you build an appropriate foundation of aerobic support and neuromuscular fitness and then mix these two ingredients together in the proper ratio. All of the training you do throughout the entire training cycle, beginning with the very first workout, should be oriented toward the goal of achieving specific endurance for your next peak race. In other words, every workout should have a specific-endurance rationale.

This does not mean every workout should be performed at or near your goal race pace. Slow recovery runs, maximal-effort hill sprints, and many other kinds of workouts that do not closely approximate the demands of racing have their place in the process of developing the capacity to meet the specific demands of racing. But what you must avoid is the common mistake of losing sight of how a particular type of training will contribute to the development of specific endurance and consequently doing too much or too little of it. For example, some runners unconsciously substitute the goal of improving their VO_2max for the goal of achieving specific endurance and therefore do too much VO_2max training (such as three-minute intervals). While VO_2max is closely associated with race performance, it is not a stand-in for race performance. Thus, by overemphasizing VO_2max training, you might fail to develop other fitness qualities that are also needed to achieve specific endurance and as a result fail to achieve your race time goal despite attaining a higher VO_2max.

Specific-Endurance Workouts

I draw a distinction between workouts that function to develop either the aerobic-support foundation or the neuromuscular-fitness foundation for specific endurance and workouts whose purpose is to develop specific endurance on top of the combined foundation of aerobic support and neuromuscular fitness. Specific-endurance workouts are workouts that aim to increase efficiency and/or fatigue resistance at or near the runner's goal race pace for a specific race distance. To qualify as a specific-endurance session, the workout must emphasize running efforts within a pace range between 10 percent slower and 10 percent faster than goal race pace. Workouts performed outside this pace range, while beneficial, are not close enough to race pace to stimulate the specific physiological adaptations that will maximize efficiency and fatigue resistance at race pace.

Let's say your peak-race goal is to break 37 minutes for 10K. Therefore your goal race pace is 5:58 per mile. A pace of 6:34 per mile is 10 percent slower than this goal race pace; a pace of 5:22 per mile is 10 percent faster. So your specific-endurance workout pace range, if your goal is to run a sub-37:00 10K, would be 6:34 to 5:22 per mile.

The closer you get to your peak race, the more your specific-endurance pace range should narrow. During the introductory and fundamental periods of training, I like to use the full 10-percent-slower-to-10-percent-faster range. In the late fundamental period and sharpening period, I narrow the range down to 3 or 4 percent above and below goal race pace. Maximizing time spent running very near your goal pace in the final weeks of training will maximize your efficiency and fatigue resistance at that pace.

Depending on the distance of your peak race, some workouts may serve as both specific-endurance and speed-interval workouts, or as both specific-endurance and threshold workouts. For example, a 5K runner who performs a set of intervals at 3K pace is really doing both a speed-interval workout and a specific-endurance workout, as 3K pace is only 4 to 5 percent faster than 5K race pace for most runners. Similarly, a threshold workout at half-marathon pace also counts as specific-endurance training for a runner preparing for a peak race at the half-marathon distance.

Because the adaptive running system aims to develop runners with well-rounded fitness, I advise all runners to perform a certain amount of training at every pace level between an easy jog and a full sprint, regardless of the distance of their peak race. Runners training for a 5K peak race should do some marathon-pace running, runners training for a marathon should do some 5K-pace running, and so forth. Thus, different runners may use the same workout in different ways, and a workout that serves primarily as a specific-endurance workout for one runner will serve a different purpose for another runner. For example, a 10K runner might run $4 \times 2K$ at 10K pace with 1-minute active recoveries as a specific-endurance workout in the late fundamental period or sharpening period. A 5K runner might do the same workout with slightly longer active recoveries as an aerobic-support workout.

As explained in previous chapters, aerobic-support workouts become more and more specific throughout the training cycle, primarily by emphasizing faster and faster pace levels. At the same time, muscle-training workouts, and in particular speed-interval workouts, become more and more race-specific throughout the training cycle by emphasizing longer, slower (but still fast) efforts and by becoming more integrated with specific-endurance training. Meanwhile, specific-endurance training progresses throughout the training cycle by emphasizing progressively longer efforts at goal pace and by reducing the duration of recovery periods between goal-pace intervals. Thus, in the sharpening period of training—the final few weeks before your peak race—there is a convergence in these three separate threads of your training, such that your three hardest workouts of the week emphasize efforts at or relatively near race pace.

Specific-endurance training culminates in a single workout that constitutes your most race-specific workout, which is performed 15 to 10 days before your peak race. This workout puts the finishing touches on your development of specific endurance and demonstrates your ability to achieve your peak-race goal time (provided you are able to sustain the appropriate pace throughout the workout). Table 5.1 presents suggested peak-level specific-endurance workouts for three categories of runners at the four popular road-race distances.

For 5K and 10K runners, these workouts should be more or less the same for runners of all ability levels, because the distances are relatively short, so that a low-key competitive runner can handle a highly race-specific 5K or 10K workout as well as a highly competitive runner can. (What makes the highly trained runner's version of the workout harder, in absolute terms, is that it is most likely run at a faster pace.) But at the longer distances—half-marathon and marathon—the formats representing the most appropriate peak-level specific-endurance workouts begin to diverge for runners at different training levels. For less-competitive runners, merely covering these longer distances is a much greater challenge than it is for highly competitive runners, for whom it is the speed they wish to sustain over that distance that represents the greater challenge.

For example, for a low-key competitive marathon runner, there is little or no difference between "just finish" pace for the marathon and race pace. But a highly competitive marathon runner might be able to easily "jog" a marathon at a pace that's one or two minutes per mile slower than his or her goal race pace for the event. Thus, the best peak-level specific-endurance workout for a low-key competitive runner is an easy run of 20 to 22 miles, whereas for a highly competitive runner it might be somewhat shorter, but far more aggressive pace-wise.

The following table presents suggested peak-level specific-endurance workouts for three categories of runners at the four popular road-race distances.

Table 5.1 Suggested Peak-Level Specific-Endurance Workouts			
	Category of Runner		
Peak-Race Distance	Low-Key Competitive	Competitive	Highly Competitive
5K	5 × 1K @ goal pace w/2-min. jog recoveries	5 × 1K @ goal pace w/90-sec. jog recoveries	5 × 1K @ 5K pace w/1-min. jog recoveries
10K	4 × 2K @ 10K pace w/1-min. jog recoveries	4 × 2K @ 10K pace + 1K @ maximum effort w/1-min. jog recoveries	4 × 2K @ 10K pace + 1K @ maximum effort w/1-min. jog recoveries
Half-Marathon	6 × 1 mile @ half-marathon pace w/2-min. jog recoveries	4 × 3K @ half-marathon pace w/90-sec. jog recoveries	3 × 5K @ half-marathon pace w/90-sec. jog recoveries
Marathon	20–22 miles easy	10 miles easy 10 miles @ marathon pace	45 min. easy + 20K: 1K on/1K off On = marathon goal pace Off = marathon pace + 5–10 sec./mile

Progression of Specific-Endurance Training

Specific-endurance workouts performed in the early part of the training cycle are necessarily different from the peak-level workouts shown in Table 5.1, which are almost as challenging as the peak race itself, because they require that the runner cover the full race distance or something close to it at race pace with minimal recovery opportunity, so that the runner must be already near his or her peak fitness level to complete them. When you introduce specific-endurance training in the introductory period, it should take the form of short, approximate efforts whose purpose is mainly to get your body accustomed to the feel of race pace. For 5K, 10K, and half-marathon runners, these efforts will most likely take the form of fartlek intervals. Marathon runners will start with a short (perhaps 10-minute) marathon-pace progression at the end of a long run.

From this point, specific-endurance training will progress toward peak level in four ways. First, specific-endurance efforts will move closer to your exact goal pace. For example, a 10K runner might do his first session of specific-endurance intervals at his current estimated 10K pace and later move up to his goal 10K pace. Second, the amount of specific-endurance running performed in a single workout will increase. For example, a half-marathon runner might advance from a workout comprising a 70-minute easy run plus a 10-minute hard progression (at roughly half-marathon pace) to a threshold run featuring 2×15 minutes @ half-marathon pace with a 2-minute active recovery (i.e., jogging) between threshold efforts. (The lion's share of specific-endurance training for half-marathon runners should occur within the context of threshold runs in the fundamental and sharpening periods.)

Third, race-pace efforts will become more extended. For example, a 10K runner might move from 1K intervals at 10K pace to 2K intervals at 10K pace. And lastly, the recovery opportunities between race-pace efforts will be shortened or, in the case of some marathon-specific workouts, performed at a faster pace. For example, a marathon runner might advance from (a) a workout including $10 \times 1K$ "on"/1K "off," in which the "on" segments are run 10 seconds per mile faster than goal marathon pace and the "off" segments are run one minute per mile slower than marathon pace to (b) one in which the "on" segments are run at goal marathon pace and the "off" segments are run just 30 seconds per mile slower.

These four patterns of progression for specific-endurance training may be used in any order from workout to workout and even simultaneously, as long as the overall challenge level does not increase too quickly from one session to the next. For example, a 5K runner might run 6×600 meters at her current 5K pace with 2-minute active recoveries in one specific-endurance workout, and in the next one run 5×800 meters at her goal 5K pace with 90-second active recoveries. In this example, the total amount of race-pace running, the duration of race-pace efforts, and the actual pace of the efforts have all increased slightly, while the recovery opportunities have been reduced.

Another sort of progression pattern that is often manifest in my application of specific-endurance training is a movement from workouts that integrate specific-endurance training with other types of training (anaerobic hill repetitions, speed intervals, threshold progressions) to workouts that focus squarely on race-pace training. For example, a 5K runner might advance from a $2 \times$ (6-minute, 5-minute, 4-minute, 3-minute, 2-minute, 1-minute) ladder interval workout, in which intervals are run between 10K pace and 1,500-meter pace, to a workout comprising 5 × 800 meters at 5K to 3K pace. While I do, in fact, use multi-pace workouts that include race-pace running throughout the training cycle, because they are an effective means of administering small doses of lower-priority training intensities, my reliance on them decreases as the training cycle unfolds. The ladder workout example I just cited might be a runner's primary specific-endurance workout in a training week occurring in the early fundamental period, whereas it might be used to provide a second dose of specific-endurance training plus a little speed work in the sharpening period, perhaps three days after an exclusively race-pace interval session.

It's not important that your specific-endurance workout progressions be totally systematic. What's important is that your first bit of specific-endurance training be appropriate to your current fitness level, that your subsequent specific-endurance workouts become a little more race-specific from session to session, and that your peak-level specific-endurance workout be challenging and specific enough to all but ensure that you achieve your peak-race time goal, provided you complete the workout at the required level. But it's okay to be somewhat creative and spontaneous in developing each particular specific-endurance workout format as you go.

Let's now look at some examples of specific-endurance workout progressions for each of the four popular road-race distances. These examples are not intended to be used as actual training plans to be followed exactly as they are written. Rather, they are intended simply to provide concrete examples of how specific-endurance training should evolve over the course of a training cycle. The 12-workout sequence for each distance does not represent an exhaustive list of every specific-endurance workout you might do in a given training cycle; it is only a selection of benchmarks or stepping-stones that you might hit en route to a peak race, along with other specific-endurance workouts that are not listed but whose design might be inferred by imagining a session that represents a halfway point between any two sequential workouts on the list. This is especially true for the marathon plan. While 12 specific-endurance workouts might be sufficient to prepare a runner with a decent base-fitness level for a peak-level 5K performance, a marathon runner would almost certainly require more.

These tables also should not be taken to imply that one must always do one specific-endurance workout per week every week throughout the training cycle. While it's best to

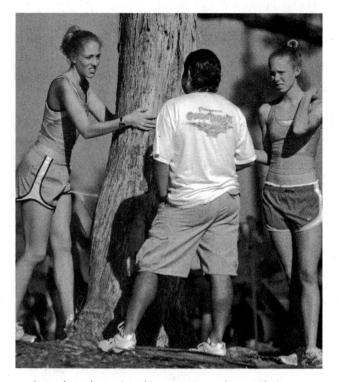

A good coach monitors his runners to make sure their fitness is moving in the direction of race-specificity. As a self-coached runner you must do the same for yourself.
© Alison Wade

do some race-pace running each week, your major specific-endurance sessions may be spread out by as much as 10 days in the foundation period. The sample adaptive training plans in Chapter 12 will give you a more complete picture of appropriate specific-endurance workout progressions in the total training context.

Finally, most of the workouts laid out in the following tables are appropriate only for runners at a certain level of fitness and training. In creating these sample progressions, I had in mind hypothetical runners averaging 35 to 45 miles per week for 5K, 40 to 50 miles per week for 10K, 50 to 60 miles per week for the half-marathon, and 55 to 65 miles per week for the marathon.

Specific-Endurance Training for 5K

Specific-endurance training for the 5K is fairly straightforward, because every 5K runner should aim toward the same peak-level 5K specific-endurance workout: 5 × 1K @ 5K goal pace with 1-minute jog recoveries. All of the preceding specific-endurance workouts in the training cycle should be structured and arranged to ensure that you are able to complete the peak-level workout at your goal pace.

Start your 5K specific-endurance training with fartlek intervals in the 10K- to 3K-pace range in the introductory period. It's best to do one such workout per week, because it delivers a manageable dose, and most likely your only dose, of race-pace running at this stage. Progress by adding intervals, increasing the duration of intervals, and increasing the overall duration of the workout.

As fartlek interval workouts are phased out in the transition from the introductory period to the fundamental period, hill repetitions, speed intervals, and race-pace intervals are phased in. Hill repetitions prepare 5K runners to better handle the stress of challenging speed and race-pace interval sessions by building strength along with speed and specific endurance. Therefore I recommend that you do at least one hill-repetition workout before taking on your first challenging speed and/or race-pace interval workout. But you don't have to delay your first such workout until after you've completed a "block" of hill repetition sessions, as this table may seem to suggest. Just avoid doing your first very hard speed and/or race-pace interval session until after you have a couple of hill-repetition sessions in your legs.

I keep saying "speed and/or race-pace" because in the early fundamental period your specific-endurance workouts should emphasize efforts at 5K to 1,500-meter pace, a range in which 5K specific endurance blends with speed. The objective of your specific-endurance workout progression in this period is to gradually extend your speed by increasing the distance of the intervals you run at race pace and faster.

By the late fundamental period, your specific-endurance workouts should focus squarely on your goal 5K pace. Take your specific endurance to peak level by continuing to increase your interval distance to an upper limit of 1K and then cutting the jogging recovery periods between intervals down to one minute.

Fartlek Intervals 8 × 30 sec. @ 10K–3K pace
Fartlek Intervals 8 × 40 sec. @ 10K–3K pace
8 × 300m hills @ current 3K pace w/2-min. jog recoveries
8 × 400m hills @ goal 5K pace w/2-min. jog recoveries
Ladder Intervals 2 × (6 min., 5 min., 4 min., 3 min., 2 min., 1 min.) @ 10K–1,500m pace w/90-sec. jog recoveries between intervals, 2-min. walk recovery between sets
10 × 400m @ current 5K–3K pace w/2-min. jog recoveries
12 × 400m @ current 5K–3K pace w/2-min. jog recoveries

7 × 600m @ current 5K pace w/2-min. jog recoveries
5 × 800 @ goal 5K pace w/90-sec. jog recoveries
6 × 800 @ goal 5K pace w/90-sec. jog recoveries
5 × 1K @ goal 5K pace w/90-sec. jog recoveries
5 × 1K @ goal 5K pace w/1-min. jog recoveries

Specific-Endurance Training for 10K

Most competitive runners are capable of performing the same peak-level 10K specific-endurance workout, which, like the 5K peak-level specific-endurance workout, should be performed roughly 10 days before your peak race. My preferred format is 4 × 2K @ 10K goal pace with 1-minute jog recoveries plus 1K @ maximal effort. This session is actually a little tougher than the slightly more race-specific alternative: 5 × 2K @ 10K goal pace. The first format tells me a little more about the athlete's race readiness, too, because the maximal-effort 1K finish shows exactly how much fuel is left in the tank after 8K of running at 10K goal pace.

The specific-endurance training that precedes either one of these peak-level workouts must gradually prepare you to complete it successfully. As with the 5K, the progression starts with fartlek intervals in the introductory period. These may be more numerous and slightly slower than they are for a 5K runner, to make the workout a little more 10K-specific, but it doesn't matter much.

You have the option to perform one or more hill-repetition workouts at the beginning of the fundamental period to build more specific strength before you take on your first hard specific-endurance interval workout at the track. If you choose to do some hill repetitions, they may be a little longer and slower than they are for a 5K runner.

The remainder of the fundamental period is devoted to extending your 10K speed. Begin with short intervals at 5K pace and then gradually increase the length of your specific efforts and slow the pace, stopping at 10K goal pace in the late fundamental period. Once you are running close to 10K in total distance at 10K goal pace in your specific-endurance workouts, shorten the active recoveries to 1 minute.

Fartlek Intervals 10 × 30 sec. @ 10K–3K pace
Fartlek Intervals 10 × 40 sec. @ 10K–3K pace
Fartlek Intervals 10 × 50 sec. @ 10K–3K pace
8 × 400m hills @ current 5K pace w/2-min. jog recoveries
8 × 600m hills @ current 5K pace w/2-min. jog recoveries
8 × 800m @ current 10K–5K pace w/2-min. jog recoveries
8 × 1K @ current 10K pace w/2-min. jog recoveries
8 × 1K @ goal 10K pace w/90-sec. jog recoveries
6 × 1 mile @ goal 10K pace w/90-sec. jog recoveries
5 × 2K @ goal 10K pace w/90-sec. jog recoveries
4 × 2K @ goal 10K pace + 1K max effort w/1-min. jog recoveries

Specific-Endurance Training for the Half-Marathon

The half-marathon is similar to the 10K in one way, but different in another. On the one hand, most competitive runners are able to run a half-marathon at a pace that's only 15 to 20 seconds per mile slower than their 10K race pace. On the other hand, the half-marathon is more than twice the distance of the 10K and presents a significantly greater endurance challenge.

Due to its unique nature, the half-marathon demands a different approach to specific-endurance training than shorter races. Specifically, when training for a half-marathon peak race, you should distribute your specific-endurance training stimuli among three separate types of workouts: specific-endurance interval sessions, threshold workouts, and long runs. While 5K and 10K runners perform threshold workouts and long runs as well, half-marathon runners must rely on these workouts more heavily to develop their specific endurance, whereas for 5K and 10K runners these slower workouts serve almost entirely to develop aerobic support.

Half-marathon runners should approach specific-endurance intervals in more or less the same way as 10K runners. The only difference is that their last few specific-endurance interval workouts should focus on half-marathon goal pace and should include more total goal-pace running. Threshold runs should include efforts at marathon pace (or slightly faster), half-marathon pace, and between half-marathon pace and 10K pace, with the total amount of threshold running in each session and especially the amount of half-marathon-pace running gradually increasing. In the sharpening period, specific-endurance workouts and threshold workouts are almost indistinguishable for the half-marathon runner.

Long runs, meanwhile, must first establish the basic endurance needed to easily cover the half-marathon distance and then develop the capacity to cover this distance at faster and faster speeds. For the low-mileage runner, long runs are really the primary specific-endurance workout, because at the start of the training cycle such a runner might not be able to run 13.1 miles at *any* pace.

The following table shows only the specific-endurance intervals progression. It is fairly challenging and is appropriate only for runners who are capable of at least jogging 13.1 miles at the beginning of the training cycle and who are willing and able to train at least 45 miles per week, on average.

Fartlek Intervals 10 × 40 sec. @ 10K–3K pace
Fartlek Intervals 10 × 50 sec. @ 10K–3K pace
1 hour easy + 4 × 600m uphill @ 5K–3K pace
6 × 800m @ current 5K–3K pace w/2-min. jog recoveries
5 × 1K @ 5K pace w/2-min. jog recoveries
Ladder Intervals 2 × (3K @ half-marathon pace, 2K @ current 10K pace, 1K @ current 5K pace w/2-min. jog recoveries)
6 × 1 mile @ current 10K pace
4 × 2K @ goal 10K pace + 1K max effort w/90-sec. jog recoveries
8 × 1 mile @ goal half-marathon pace w/90-sec. jog recoveries
4 × 3K @ goal half-marathon pace w/90-sec. jog recoveries
3 × 5K @ goal half-marathon pace w/90-sec. jog recoveries

Specific-Endurance Training for the Marathon

Everything is different when it comes to the marathon, and specific-endurance training is no exception. In the adaptive running system, specific-endurance training for the marathon occurs primarily within the context of long runs. Because the endurance challenge of the marathon is so great, the first priority of your long runs is to develop the endurance required to cover the full marathon distance comfortably. The next priority is to gradually increase the pace you can sustain over that distance, up to your goal marathon race pace.

If your marathon goal is not just to finish but to achieve a certain finishing time, begin doing a small amount of goal-marathon-pace running in your Sunday long runs in the very first weeks of the training cycle. A 10-minute marathon-pace progression at the end of an otherwise easy long run of manageable duration will serve to begin the process of developing efficiency at the pace you will have to sustain for 26.2 miles a few months down the road. From this starting point, gradually increase the duration of your long runs, the average pace of your long runs, and the amount of goal-pace running you do within them. You may alternate back and forth between workouts that emphasize distance covered, with less faster running, and long runs that emphasize the amount of faster running you do, with less total distance covered.

The best format for specific-endurance long runs in the late fundamental period and sharpening period is a very long "warm-up" of 45 minutes to an hour followed by repeated on/off cycles of faster and slower running. In your first such workout, run the "on" segments faster than marathon goal pace and the "off" segments quite a bit slower. Progress by slightly slowing down the pace of the "on" segments and significantly increasing the pace of the "off" segments.

Your peak-level specific-endurance workout must be both very long and quite heavy on race-pace running, covering at least 18 miles in total distance and including at least 10 miles at goal pace. You should also do at least one long run whose total duration is equal to your marathon goal time (unless your goal is just to finish, in which case you should try to do at least one 20-mile run).

As a supplement to the specific-endurance training you accomplish within the context of long runs, you can also do some long threshold runs, usually scheduled for Tuesday or Friday, which focus on extending marathon speed and slightly faster pace levels over longer and longer distances. The following table incorporates a few such workouts, which you can identify by their inclusion of some running at half-marathon pace.

1-hour easy run + 10 min. uphill @ goal marathon pace
30 min. easy 10 min. @ goal marathon pace 1 min. easy 10 min. @ current half-marathon pace 1 min. easy 10 min. @ current half-marathon/10K pace
90 min. easy + 20 min. @ goal marathon pace
30 min. easy 15 min. @ current half-marathon pace 3 min. easy 15 min. @ current half-marathon pace 10 min. easy
2 hours easy + 20 min. @ goal marathon pace
30 min. easy 15 min. @ goal marathon pace 1 min. easy 15 min. @ current half-marathon pace 1 min. easy 10 min. @ current half-marathon/10K pace 5 min. easy
10K easy + 10 × 1 min. on/1 min. off On = goal marathon pace − 10 sec./mile Off = goal marathon pace + 1 min./mile
2 hours easy 20 min. @ marathon pace + 20 sec./mile 20 min. @ goal marathon pace
10K easy + 10 × 1K on/1K off On = goal marathon pace − 5 sec. per mile Off = goal marathon pace + 45 sec./mile
1 hour easy + 5 × 2K on/1K off On = goal marathon pace Off = goal marathon pace + 30 sec./mile
1 hour easy + 4 × 3K on/1K off On = goal marathon pace Off = goal marathon pace + 15 sec./mile

Specific-Endurance Tests

A specific-endurance test or "spec test" is a workout designed to assess how close your current fitness level is to the level it will need to reach if you're going to achieve your goal race time. As I have mentioned already, developing race-specific endurance is the whole point of training. Every workout you do should move you toward this objective in some way. But it's not always easy to tell whether your race-specific fitness is improving. That's where spec tests come in.

There's a difference between improving your performance in whichever sorts of workouts you might be emphasizing in a particular phase of training and improving your specific endurance. For example, suppose you're training for a 5K. You've run a set of very fast 400m speed intervals with long recoveries each of the past three Tuesdays, and your split times have improved markedly. This is a sure sign that you're getting fitter, right? Not exactly. The only thing you know for sure is that you're getting better at running that workout. Without those recovery periods, you might find that you fatigue very quickly, even at a slower pace. I've seen this sort of thing happen many times.

There are only two ways to be certain that your specific endurance is improving. The first is to run a race. But this option is only practical for 5K and 10K runners, who can race at these distances every few weeks without overtaxing their bodies. A second option—and really the only option for half-marathon and marathon runners—is to perform a very race-specific workout.

A good spec test for the 5K is the same workout you will use as your peak-level specific-endurance workout: 5 × 1K @ 5K pace. The only difference is that the recovery periods are longer—2 minutes instead of 1 minute. Try to sustain your goal race pace throughout all five intervals—how close you come to doing so, or how easily you are able to do so, will reveal the current state of your specific endurance for the 5K.

I'm not going to give you some magical formula that will tell you exactly what your split times for this workout should be in relation to your goal pace at various points in the training cycle. Your gut will tell you. Just do the workout, look at your split times, compare them to your goal pace, and consider how much training you have left to do before your goal race, and you'll have a feeling for whether your training is on track.

Do the spec test (or run a 5K tune-up race, if you prefer) every five or six weeks. Naturally, you will want to see a certain amount of improvement each time you repeat it. When your level of improvement is disappointing, you know it's time to make a change in your training. I'll discuss how to make such changes in chapter 8.

My preferred spec test for the 10K is also identical to the peak-level 10K specific-endurance workout, save for longer rest periods. Run 4 × 2K @ 10K goal pace + 1K @ maximal effort with 3-minute jog recoveries (instead of 1-minute jog recoveries). As with the 5K spec test, do this 10K test (or run a 10K tune-up race) once every five or six weeks to see how close your fitness level is to your desired peak level.

The half-marathon requires a different sort of diagnostic test. There are two options, actually. The first is what I usually call an aerobic test, and it requires a heart-rate monitor. Step one is to come up with a ballpark estimate of your current half-marathon race pace in the context of doing your normal workouts involving efforts at your current half-marathon race pace. Wear a heart-rate monitor during these workouts and note the heart rate that is associated with your current half-marathon race pace. This is your half-marathon heart rate, which will not change much between now and your goal race. What will change is the pace you can sustain at this heart rate. You'll have achieved peak-race fitness if and when your half-marathon heart rate and your goal half-marathon pace match·up.

Now you're ready for your aerobic spec test. Go to the local track and, after a thorough warm-up, run for 20 to 30 minutes at your half-marathon heart rate. Stop after the designated test duration has elapsed and note how far you've run. Use the time and distance data to calculate your pace. Repeat this test once every five or six weeks. You should move closer to your goal half-marathon pace each time.

If you don't use a heart-rate monitor, you can perform a somewhat more objective alternative half-marathon spec test. Go to the local track, warm up thoroughly, and start the test. Instead of using heart rate to set your pace at your current half-marathon level, use perceived effort—that is, simply run at the fastest pace you feel you could sustain through an entire half-marathon. Run exactly 4 miles (16 laps + 40 yards) at this effort level. Don't take any split times, as doing so might affect your pacing. Stop at 4 miles and use your time to calculate your pace. Repeat this test once every five or six weeks. You should move closer to your goal half-marathon pace each time.

There is really no way to perform an effective specific-endurance test for the marathon. Performance in the marathon is almost always determined by what happens in the final 10K, after 20 miles of race-pace running are completed. Either you hold pace or you fall apart. Challenging marathon-pace workouts can give you a good sense of your capacity to hold your goal marathon pace for 20 miles, but no workout can tell you what will happen in the decisive closing 10K on race day. The best you can do is look for consistent improvement as you follow your specific-endurance workout progression throughout the training cycle.

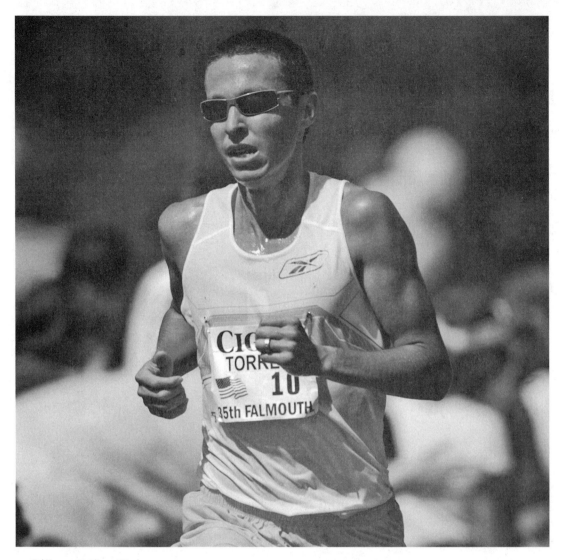

Ed Torres © Alison Wade

Runner Profile: Edwardo Torres

Edwardo Torres is the twin brother of Jorge Torres, whom I also coach. Ed has often run

in the shadow of Jorge, not so much because Jorge is more talented as because Ed has

struggled with recurrent injuries (several stress fractures and bursitis in his hip) and the

doubts and frustration that his frequent breakdowns have caused. When I started coaching him in 2005, Ed had never trained at a high enough level for a long enough stretch of time to achieve the sort of race performance he was capable of.

I helped Ed break free from his pattern of injury with my usual methods. He had never done any true strength and power training before I had him start doing hill sprints, which improved his strength dramatically. I also increased his running mileage substantially. Always a relatively low-mileage runner in the past, Ed initially had a hard time believing me when I insisted that consistent high mileage would *reduce* his risk of injury, provided we worked our way up the volume ladder carefully. Thankfully, he decided to trust me, and he has been able to run relatively injury-free for a while now.

In addition to working hard to increase Ed's physical strength and durability, I have also put a lot of effort into transforming his mind-set about training. Ed's disposition is such that he would rather do 70 miles a week of very hard running than 120 miles of mostly moderate running with a few carefully chosen hard running opportunities. He had to develop the attitude that running 120 to 130 miles per week was no big deal, which is the attitude of most elite marathon runners. Now that Ed has achieved this mind-set, I am confident he will soon become one of the most successful marathon runners in the United States.

Self-Assessment

6

In addition to coaching the members of the Performance Training Group, I also advise runners periodically on a less formal basis. Every now and again I receive a call or an e-mail message from a friend of a friend who asks for my help in constructing a training plan. While I really prefer to take an all-or-nothing approach to coaching runners, I get such a kick out of building training plans that I don't mind fulfilling these requests if I feel that I can truly help the runner.

Before I create a training plan for any runner that I don't know well already, I ask for certain bits of information that I will need to make sure the plan is a proper fit. My plans are always based on the general adaptive running methods described in the previous five chapters. But these general methods can be applied in countless particular ways. The right way to apply them depends on the individual's background, strengths, weaknesses, and goals. So I must gather some specific data in these areas before I can make a good plan for any runner.

As a self-coached runner, you need to consider the same factors in choosing or creating an adaptive training plan for yourself. This means that you must complete a thorough self-assessment before you start plunking workouts into a schedule. In this chapter, I'll discuss each of 10 individual factors that I consider in designing training plans for runners and explain how to use each factor in your running self-assessment and training-plan selection or design. These 10 factors are:

1. recent training

2. running experience

3. age

4. past race performances

5. short-term goal

6. injury history

7. event-specific strength and weakness

8. recovery profile

9. long-term goal

10. motivational profile

The order in which I've listed these 10 self-assessment factors is not random. They are listed according to their relative weightiness in affecting how you should train. All of the factors are important, but your recent training (factor number 1) is the consideration that should have the greatest influence on your training-program design. Your individual motivational profile (factor number 10) should have a much smaller influence.

The one ranking in this list that is somewhat forced is that of the short-term goal. In a sense, your short-term goal should be your first consideration, since your training will necessarily be completely different if your short-term goal is to finish your first marathon than it will be if your short-term goal is to set a new 5K personal record. But since the first four factors—recent training, running experience, age, and personal best times—are essential considerations in establishing an appropriate short-term goal, I've listed the short-term goal as the fifth factor. So, without further ado, let's look at each factor individually.

1. Recent Training

The training you've done over the past two years, and especially within the past 12 months, is, for better or worse, the foundation for the training you will do in your next training cycle. There are specific possible inadequacies in your recent training that you should look for and attempt to address in planning your next training cycle:

• Inadequate mileage

• Inadequate balance

• Inadequate specific-endurance training

More likely than not, you'll need to run more miles than you've done recently to improve as quickly as possible. But if you try to drastically increase your running mileage, you'll probably get injured. So, if you're ready and willing to train harder in your next training cycle than you did in your previous one, plan to increase your average and peak weekly training mileage by as much as, but no more than, 50 percent, and ease into it.

In chapter 3, I presented a table that provides average weekly training-mileage guidelines for five categories of runner preparing for peak races at four distances. Refer back to this table when you begin your self-assessment process. If your recent average weekly running volume was lower than the recommended range for your category and event, plan to bump it up into the optimal range. If you're ready to move up to the next category, then plan an average weekly volume that falls within the optimal range for that category, unless it's more than 50 percent more than your recent weekly volume, in which case you should increase your weekly running volume by 50 percent.

Don't feel obligated to increase your running mileage if you are unable or unwilling to devote more time to training. There are other ways to improve besides running more.

In addition to the amount of training, you must also consider the types of training you've done recently. One of the first things I look for in the past training of runners who begin working with me is lack of balance, and one of the most important things I try to do in designing a training program for a new athlete is to create more balance. A well-balanced training program should have the following basic elements:

- Easy runs
- Long runs
- Steep hill sprints
- Moderate progression runs
- Threshold runs
- Speed/specific-endurance intervals
- Strides and drills

Each of these elements should be present to some degree in your training more or less throughout the training cycle. If any of them has been absent in your recent training, you must add it. Of course, the aim is not to achieve a perfect balance. Certain types of training should have a larger or smaller overall presence in your training, depending on your goals and other factors. And your training priorities should always evolve from the extremes toward specificity throughout the training cycle. But I rarely come across a runner who has adequate balance in his or her training, and chances are you're no exception to this pattern.

Be aware that lack of balance may also result from doing too much of a particular type of training. If there's any specific type of training that you have "done to death" over the past two years, you should probably deemphasize it. For example, let's suppose you're a 5K specialist and in every training cycle you do at least eight workouts featuring 600-meter intervals at roughly 3K pace, because that's what your high school coach had you do to prepare for 5K cross-country races. This type of training certainly can be beneficial for 5K race performance, and I would not hesitate to have someone who's never done it start doing it, but in your case it will be better to move away from it to some degree because the training stimulus is too familiar to trigger any more improvement.

Also, review your recent training for workout types that you just don't seem to have gotten much out of. Often these workouts are the same ones that have been done to death. In any case, they, too, should probably be deemphasized. For example, let's suppose you're a veteran marathon runner who's done more easy 16- to 24-mile long runs than you can remember, and recently you've felt that this type of workout is not the endurance booster it used to be for you. (Or, put another way, you seem to get all the endurance you're going to get from a very small number of such workouts.) In your next training cycle, you should reduce the number of easy long runs you do and add more moderately long to long runs at faster speeds to stimulate new fitness adaptations.

Finally, look at the possibility of increasing the amount of specific work—that is, work at or very near your goal race pace—in planning your next training cycle. As we develop as runners, we become less responsive to general training and increasingly able to capitalize on greater amounts of specific training. Unless you have overemphasized specific training in the past, you should look to gently increase the amount of specific work you perform in your next training cycle compared to recent cycles. Runners who train for half-marathons and marathons, I find, are those most likely to underutilize specific training and thus to benefit most from boosting it.

2. Running Experience

The overall amount of running experience you have and the nature of that experience should have a profound influence in shaping your next training cycle. Beginning runners should focus on establishing a solid foundation for their future development as runners by training the extremes—that is, by focusing heavily on developing basic aerobic fitness with moderate-intensity runs of various lengths and basic neuromuscular fitness with very short, very high-intensity efforts on hills and on the track. This training approach will develop the beginning runner's fitness level as rapidly as any alternative and will lay the best foundation for further development.

As the seasons and years go by, assuming you train sensibly, your training should evolve first by adding layer upon layer to this foundation through increasing mileage and more challenging aerobic workouts, including longer long runs, and also through more challenging high-intensity muscle training. As these types of training begin to reach a point of diminishing returns, gradually shift your focus toward specific-endurance training for your primary race event.

The longer you continue training for competitive performance in the sport of distance running, the more your overall training mix should move away from general training at the extremes and the more it should focus on specific endurance and optimal aerobic support. The following table provides general parameters to guide this developmental process.

Continuous Running Experience	Major Training Priorities
1–4 Years	• Gradually build easy mileage • Increase long run distance • Hill sprints • Hill intervals • Short intervals (including fartlek) • Minimal specific-endurance training
5–7 Years	• Continue building mileage • Faster long runs • Threshold runs • Tougher speed workouts • Gradually increase specific-endurance training
8+ Years	• Maximize mileage • Very hard long runs • Challenging threshold runs • Increasingly emphasize specific-endurance training

3. Age

The age of a runner can be difficult to dissociate from his or her running experience. You very seldom encounter a veteran 12-year-old runner, while most runners in their 50s have been at it for a decade or more. Nevertheless, age is at least a semi-independent factor to consider in planning a training cycle.

Runners in their late teens and early 20s have a much greater margin for error in their training than older runners have. Virtually any type of training that does not injure them or result in chronic overtraining fatigue will improve their fitness and performance. Like all runners, they will derive the greatest benefit from the most appropriate training, but young runners are typically able to get a greater benefit from less specific and even borderline-irrelevant training than older runners. Nevertheless, runners of every age should train as appropriately as possible.

Due to their strong recovery capacity, young runners generally do not need to train as easy on their easy days as older runners do. If you're between 15 and 25 years old, you can probably train at least moderately hard every time you run, assuming you have an active background, if not a running background. You can reserve the very slow recovery runs that older runners depend on for those rare days when you feel especially lousy. However, by the same token, young runners cannot expect to train quite as hard in their key workouts as more experienced runners in their late 20s and early 30s. It takes years of consistent training to reach the point where you are able to tackle the toughest workouts you will ever do, and no runner under the age of 26 has this foundation. It's okay to do some gut-busting training sessions when you're young, but always hold back a little in planning these workouts. Take the long view, and draw patience from the knowledge that those epic track sessions and long threshold runs you dream of doing are waiting for you just a few seasons down the road.

If you suspect I don't apply this wisdom with the young runners I coach, guess again. Dathan Ritzenhein (age 25 at the time of this writing) has chafed to train harder than I've allowed him to since the day he started working with me, but I have held him back with a firm hand. Each year I let him loose a little more—not as much as he would like, but enough to make a difference. And Dathan will be the first to admit that this imposed restraint has been good for him. He feels stronger all the time, and he never feels overwhelmed by his training the way he sometimes did before he began working with me, when there was no one to hold him back.

The period between the mid- to late 20s and the mid- to late 30s constitutes another stage in a runner's development that requires a slightly different approach to training. At this time, your capacity to recover from hard training is decreasing, so you need to take it very easy on your easy days to fully absorb your most recent hard session and get ready for your next one. On the other hand, if you've been training consistently for at least a few years now, you can handle harder workouts than you could as a whippersnapper, because your body has changed dramatically in response to all of that past training. Your muscles, bones, joints, and neuroendocrine system are now, in a concrete sense, far better designed for hard training than they were when you were younger.

Somewhere between the ages of 40 and 45 a third stage in the development of a runner begins. In this stage, it is extremely important to get the most bang for your buck from workouts and to eliminate as much waste as possible from your training. The majority of your key workouts should be very race-specific. There's not much to be gained from general training anymore. Your body has adapted to so many different training stimuli over so many years that there are few remaining stimuli that are capable of triggering fresh fitness adaptations, so you have to choose very carefully. You're a long way from those early days when virtually anything that got your heart rate up made you a better runner. On the positive side, your years of training and racing have taught you many things about yourself as a runner, and you can use this knowledge to select just the right alterations to your training approach that will keep you moving forward.

There should be few or no "junk miles" in your training after age 40. Accumulated wear and tear on your body has probably already put you past the point of being able to set new personal records, and continuing to fill your schedule with a lot of basic aerobic runs will do more harm, in the form of additional wear and tear, than it will do good, in the form of new aerobic adaptations. You're better off doing just three or four focused sessions per week in the muscle-training, aerobic-support (with an emphasis on threshold runs), and specific-endurance categories, and doing strength training or cardiovascular cross-training on the other days.

Masters runners also need to be careful with speed work (training at 5K race pace and faster). The muscles and connective tissues have lost elasticity by this age, making them more susceptible to strain during high-speed running. As a masters runner, you should do as much speed work as you can safely handle, and as is relevant to your event goals, but be prepared to find that you cannot safely handle very much. Adjusting your speed work for your age does not necessarily or exclusively mean doing less of it, though. You can also move some or all of it onto hills, which will reduce tissue strain at higher intensities, or you can simply slow it down a little—replacing 1,500-meter-pace intervals with 3,000-meter-pace intervals, for example.

The following three tables provide an example of how a runner's training might evolve over the course of his or her running career, based on the guidelines I've given. Each table represents a week of foundation-period training for a short-term goal of running a 34:00 10K at a specific age: 24, 34, and 44.

Age 24 (Total miles: 66 +/−)		
Sunday	2 hours easy/moderate	
Monday	45 min. easy + 10 × 8-sec. short hill sprint	
Tuesday	30 min. moderate + 5 × 3-min. hill climbs w/recovery jog back down	
Wednesday	70 min. moderate	
Thursday	45 min. moderate	
Friday	AM: 20 min. moderate	PM: 40 min. w/20-min. @ threshold pace
Saturday	50 min. moderate	

Age 34 (Total miles: 58 +/−)	
Sunday	1 hour 40 min. easy/moderate
Monday	45 min. easy + 10 × 8-sec. short hill sprint
Tuesday	20-min. warm-up Ladder intervals: 6 min., 5 min., 4 min., 3 min., 2 min., 1 min. w/3-min. active recoveries 10-min. cool-down
Wednesday	60 min. easy
Thursday	45 min. easy
Friday	20-min. warm-up 2 × 3K @ 10K goal pace w/3-min. active recoveries 10-min. cool-down
Saturday	40 min. easy

Age 44 (Total miles: 48 +/−)	
Sunday	80 min. w/ 20 min. @ threshold pace
Monday	Off or X-train
Tuesday	20-min. warm-up 8 × 3 min. @ 10K pace w/1-min. active recoveries 20-min. cool-down
Wednesday	60 min. moderate
Thursday	40 min. moderate
Friday	20-min. warm-up 5 × 3-min. hill intervals @ 5K intensity, w/recovery jog back down 20-min. cool-down
Saturday	Off or X-train

4. Past Race Performances

Your past race performances provide valuable information that you can use to guide your future training. In particular, I suggest that you consider your very best race performances and the training that preceded them. Try to identify those aspects of your training that were most responsible for your success in these events, and incorporate them into your future training.

What was different about the training that preceded your lifetime best 5K, 10K, half-marathon, and/or marathon that was different from the training that preceded less satisfying race performances? Were you running more mileage? Getting more recovery between hard workouts? Doing a better job of staying injury-free? Hitting the track more often?

Whichever training patterns you identify as being most responsible for your greatest racing successes, be sure that your next training plan also includes them, even if you're targeting a race of a different distance. Assuming you have at least a modest amount of past racing experience to draw upon, your best-ever race performances will provide a good indication of the general training patterns to which you respond best. Of course, they may also tell you what your ideal race distance is, but even if you are now training for a longer or shorter race, this information is relevant, because the training patterns that get you into the best shape at any specific race distance are likely to also help you get into the best possible shape for other race distances, assuming you make commonsense adjustments for the different speed and endurance demands of your current race focus.

There is really very little difference in the type of fitness that is needed to run your best 5K and the type that is needed to run your best marathon, or any intermediate distance. (Elite male runners run less than 45 seconds per mile slower in the marathon than they do in the 5K.) If you're in shape to run your best time at any distance between 5K and the marathon, you won't be far off optimal shape for any other distance. In preparing for a race of any distance, you can't go wrong by relying on training practices that are proven to prepare you optimally for any other race distance. Simply contextualize the training differently based on the specific distance of your next peak race.

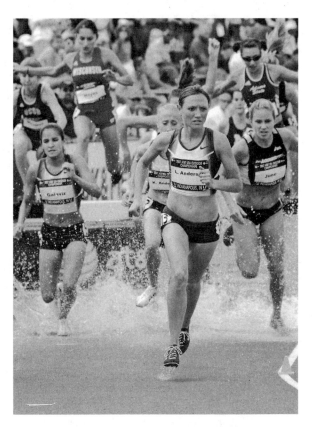

Your past race performances provide valuable information you can use in designing your next training plan. © Alison Wade

I am not suggesting that you simply duplicate your past training in any degree of detail. If your best race ever was a 5K you ran in college 10 years ago, don't go and contact your college coach to have him e-mail you his favorite track workouts. What I am suggesting is that you reuse general training patterns that seem to have worked well for you in the past.

For example, suppose your best past race performance was a half-marathon in which you set a big surprise personal record (PR). When you consider how the training that preceded it was different from the training that preceded less-satisfying half-marathons, you recall that when you set your PR you were focusing on shorter races (5K's and 10K's), and you raced the half-marathon as a lark, only because a friend talked you into it, whereas all of your other half-marathons were run as tune-up races during marathon-focused training. This information may tell you that you respond best to a training approach that emphasizes high-intensity workouts and slightly deemphasizes long runs and overall mileage as compared to what might work best for other runners.

If your past racing experience is limited, you will of course be limited in your ability to use your history of competitive performances to identify the types of training to which you respond best. In this case, just use the other nine self-assessment factors discussed in this chapter to customize your next training cycle. After you complete the peak race in which this next training cycle culminates, you'll have more material to use to determine which particular training patterns work best for you.

5. Short-Term Goal

Your short-term goal is a performance goal you wish to achieve in your next peak race. These goals almost always take the form of a specific finishing time in a chosen race of a certain distance on a particular date. Always set a short-term goal at least 12 weeks ahead of time. Seldom, if ever, will you need more than 24 weeks of focused preparation to achieve a short-term goal, but you can always set a short-term goal farther out if you don't intend to immediately begin focused preparation for it. The lower your current fitness level is and the longer your next peak race, the more preparation time you should allow.

Most runners with at least a couple of years' worth of racing experience are pretty good at setting realistic race time goals. All it takes is one overambitious goal resulting in disaster on race day to correct an inflated sense of one's current running abilities. If you have minimal race experience or are planning to race at an unfamiliar distance, you can use a performance equivalency calculator to help you set a time goal. Using such a calculator, you input a race time at one distance and then the program spits out predicted finishing times, or equivalent performances, at other races distances. You can find a good one at www.mcmillanrunning.com.

In any case, the purpose of setting a short-term goal is not to predict the future. You can and most likely will have to adjust your goal time based on your fitness development as the training cycle unfolds and race day draws nearer. The true purpose of setting a short-term goal is to establish parameters for the training cycle that will culminate in that peak race. The objective of your training is to develop the capacity to sustain your goal pace for the full race distance on race day. Knowing how fast and how far you have to run to achieve your goal tells you what sorts of race-specific workouts you'll need to be able to perform in the final weeks of training. Knowing the precise nature of these peak workouts—and understanding the principles of adaptive running—enables you to then determine the general progression of key workouts you will need to arrange between the start of the training cycle and the sharpening phase. These workouts must serve to establish the proper foundation of aerobic and neuromuscular fitness and then build incrementally more race-specific fitness on top of this foundation as the weeks go by.

6. Injury History

Some runners are more injury-prone than others. If you consider yourself injury-prone, I recommend that you include more hill running in your future training than you might otherwise do. In addition, you should take a more cautious approach to increasing your running mileage and increasing the volume of high-intensity running in your training.

Nearly all of the common overuse injuries that runners suffer from are caused in part by lack of strength in one or more muscles, which in turn causes joint instability. Short hill sprints boost running-specific strength and power tremendously. They subject the muscles and joint tissues to the highest levels of stress for very short periods of time, thus stimulating the greatest possible strengthening adaptations without themselves causing injuries.

I prescribe short hill sprints for all of my runners, but my injury-prone runners do more of them, usually by continuing to do hill sprints twice per week throughout the training cycle instead of moving from two sessions to one session midway through it. You can further reduce your risk of injury by moving some of your high-intensity workouts—intervals and threshold runs—from level terrain to inclines. This will reduce impact forces and joint strain while further increasing your running-specific strength.

The use of hill running as a primary injury-prevention technique seems strange to many runners, but it really works. Most of the runners I coach had terrible injury problems before they started working with me. None of them used steep hill sprints in their training prior to joining my team. Steep hill sprints subsequently became a staple for each of them. All of them have been almost completely injury-free ever since.

Running injuries most often occur during periods when the training workload (either total mileage or high-intensity running mileage) is increasing. Injury-prone runners are most likely to get hurt at such times. Thus, if you have a history of breakdowns, you may need to plan a longer training cycle with a more gradual workload ramp-up than a less injury-prone runner would need.

Once you've built up to an appropriate workload for peak fitness, I suggest that you maintain it. While it is widely assumed that high running mileage causes running injuries, it's much more accurate to say that *increasing* running mileage causes running injuries. In itself, high running mileage protects against injuries, because it produces adaptations that render the bones, muscles, and connective tissues better suited to handle repetitive impact. Maintaining a consistently high running volume helps you avoid the too-sudden increases in running volume that are much riskier, because they apply stress to the bones, muscles, and connective tissues faster than these tissues can adapt.

Consistently training at a variety of paces will also protect you against injury. Many runners make the mistake of completely phasing out high-intensity running at certain times of year. This greatly increases their chances of getting injured when they start running fast again. By including at least a small amount of high-intensity training at all times, you can minimize your risk of experiencing this particular type of injury.

7. Event-Specific Strength and Weakness

An important concept that I picked up from the "Italian school" of running, as it has come to be known, is the notion that there are two types of runner at any given race distance. First, there are those who bring more speed than endurance to a particular race distance. What this means, essentially, is that these runners would probably fare better at a shorter distance than they would at a longer one. A good example of this type of runner is Shayne Culpepper. A 5,000-meter specialist, Culpepper is packed with fast-twitch muscle fibers and therefore races successfully at 1,500 meters, too, but not at 10,000 meters.

The second type of runner at any given race distance is the type that brings more endurance than speed to the event, meaning he or she would probably perform better in a longer event than in a shorter one. A good example of this type of runner is Bob Kennedy, who was also a 5,000-meter specialist (and still holds the American record in this event, at 12:58). Kennedy is more slow-twitch and fatigue-resistant than Culpepper; consequently, he competed at a very high level at 10,000 meters, but he never even dared to enter an elite-level 1,500-meter race.

The essence of the concept is that every runner has an event-specific strength and weakness at every race distance. If you bring more speed than endurance to a given race distance, then speed is your event-specific strength and endurance your event-specific weakness at that race distance. It's important to know your event-specific strength and weakness for the race distance you plan to peak for next because it affects how you ought to train. In particular, your specific-endurance training should be based in your strength and move toward your weakness.

If speed is your event-specific strength, the objective of your specific-endurance workouts is to extend your speed over race distance. You start with short intervals at your goal race pace and then try to go longer and longer at the same pace. If you're more fatigue resistant, the goal of your specific-endurance workouts is to increase your speed over distance. Start with slow intervals of longer duration and then go faster and faster as you adapt.

Let's look at an example. Suppose you're training for a 10K peak race. First, ask yourself whether, given appropriate training, you are better suited to 5K racing or half-marathon racing. If you're not sure, simply ask yourself: If I were racing a runner of equal ability over 10K, would my best chance of beating her be to outsprint her at the finish, or to push the pace early and outlast her? If your weapon is your kick, or you're better suited to 5K racing than half-marathon racing, you should concentrate on building 10K-specific fitness by extending your speed in race-specific interval workouts. If your 10K weapon is your ability to outlast well-matched competitors, or you're better suited to half-marathon racing than 5K racing, you should focus on building 10K-specific fitness by increasing your speed over distance in race-specific interval workouts.

The table below presents a sample 12-week progression of specific-endurance workouts for a speed runner and a fatigue-resistant runner who share the goal of running a 40-minute

10K (6:26 per mile) in their next peak race. It is an oversimplified example in the sense that both progression patterns are more linear than they need to be. Ideally, each type of runner would do a few workouts from the other type's progression, and both would mix in some other types of specific-endurance workouts, such as longer hill intervals and ladder intervals. Nevertheless, the examples clearly illustrate the concept of training from one's event-specific strength toward one's event-specific weakness, which is important.

	Speed Runner	Fatigue-Resistant Runner
Week 1	6 × 400m @ 1:36 w/400m jog recoveries	4 × 1K @ 4:20 w/400m jog recoveries
Week 2	8 × 400m @ 1:36 w/400m jog recoveries	5 × 1K @ 4:16 w/400m jog recoveries
Week 3	6 × 600m @ 2:24 w/400m jog recoveries	5 × 1K @ 4:12 w/400m jog recoveries
Week 4 (Recovery week)	6 × 400m @ 1:36 w/400m jog recoveries	4 × 1K @ 4:12 w/400m jog recoveries
Week 5	4 × 800m @ 3:12 w/400m jog recoveries	4 × 1 mile @ 6:48 w/400m jog recoveries
Week 6	6 × 800m @ 3:12 w/400m jog recoveries	4 × 1 mile @ 6:42 w/400m jog recoveries
Week 7	6 × 1K @ 4:00 w/400m jog recoveries	5 × 1 mile @ 6:38 w/400m jog recoveries
Week 8 (Recovery week)	4 × 800m @ 3:12 w/400m jog recoveries	4 × 1 mile @ 6:36 w/400m jog recoveries
Week 9	4 × 1 mile @ 6:24 w/400m jog recoveries	4 × 2K @ 6:32 w/400m jog recoveries
Week 10	5 × 1 mile @ 6:24 w/400m jog recoveries	4 × 2K @ 6:28 w/400m jog recoveries
Week 11	4 × 2K @ 6:24 w/400m jog recoveries	4 × 2K @ 6:24 w/400m jog recoveries
Week 12 (Taper week)	2 × 2K @ 6:24 w/400m jog recoveries	2 × 2K @ 6:24 w/400m jog recoveries

You will have noticed that the two progressions come together with identical workouts in the final two weeks of training. This is because the two runners share the same goal. The specific fitness requirements of running a 40:00 10K are the same for all runners, regardless of type, so both speed runners and fatigue-resistant runners who share this goal should perform the most race-specific interval workout possible in the final weeks of training.

The starting points for any speed/fatigue-resistant pair of runners with a common race goal are different, and therefore so too is the path toward the endpoint, but the endpoint itself is the same.

If you're training to peak for a 5K or a half-marathon, go through the same exercise. Obviously, whether you're a speed type or an endurance type, your intervals will be shorter and faster for the 5K than they are for the 10K, and they'll be longer and slower for the half-marathon. The marathon is a case unto itself, because everyone brings more speed than endurance to this event.

8. Recovery Profile

Individual runners recover differently from different types and patterns of training. Generally, the speedier you are, the faster you'll recover from faster workouts compared to those who are more fatigue-resistant. Likewise, the more fatigue-resistant you are, the faster you'll recover from long runs relative to speed-type runners. But some runners recover from all challenging workouts (fast and long) either faster or slower than most other runners of equal ability. Typically, the higher your overall talent level and fitness level are, the faster you'll recover. The older you get, the slower you'll recover.

There are four variables you can manipulate to accommodate your personal recovery patterns (or recovery profile) when designing a training plan:

1. The number of hard workouts you do each week
2. The distribution of your hard workouts throughout the week
3. The degree of difficulty of your hard workouts
4. The amount of running you do between hard workouts

My adaptive running system uses a standard weekly distribution of key workouts that I recommend for every runner, regardless of his or her recovery profile. I believe this format is universally optimal for two reasons. First, it incorporates plenty of variety in workout types. Second, it distributes the key training stimuli throughout the week to provide maximum recovery opportunity following each of them. Here's the format:

Sunday	Monday	Tuesday	Wednesday	Thursday	Friday	Saturday
Long Run	Hill Sprints	Hard workout (speed, specific-endurance, threshold)			Hard workout (speed, specific-endurance, threshold)	

Using this workout schedule takes care of the first two variables listed above, leaving variables 3 and 4 as those you should focus on manipulating to ensure that your training schedule provides the right balance of training stress and recovery opportunity. The challenge level of your key workouts should be such that your fitness improves gradually and steadily throughout the training cycle. If your key workouts are too easy, your fitness level will not improve quickly enough to land you in peak shape for your peak race. If your key workouts are too hard, you will not recover sufficiently between key workouts to see your performance level rise from week to week. The challenge level of your key workouts needs to hit the sweet spot between these two extremes that cause fitness stagnation.

How is this done? When drawing up a training plan, be a little conservative in designing your key workouts for the first four to six weeks of training. In other words, plan key workouts that you are certain to have no difficulty completing and recovering from. If all goes well in those first four to six weeks, go ahead and raise the challenge level of your key workouts more aggressively in subsequent weeks. By keeping a log of your performances in those early key workouts and by paying attention to how your body feels during the early weeks of training, you should get a good sense of the proper rate at which to increase the challenge level of subsequent key workouts. Here's how your first six weeks of long runs might look if you take this approach:

Week 1: 7 miles easy

Week 2: 8 miles easy

Week 3: 9 miles easy

Week 4: 9.5 miles easy + 0.5-mile moderate progression

Week 5: 10 easy + 1.5-mile moderate uphill progression

Week 6: 11 miles easy + 2-mile moderate uphill progression

As for variable number 4—the amount of running you do between key workouts—the guiding principles are similar. Your general goal should be to do as much running between key workouts as you can without hampering your performance progress in these workouts. It's easy enough to make adjustments to the duration and pace of your easier runs on the fly as you proceed through a training cycle, but because easy runs make an important contribution to overall running volume, and because running volume is a crucial variable to optimize in designing a training plan, it's best to plan targets for the frequency and duration of your easy runs ahead of time.

These targets will need to depend on your knowledge of your recovery profile. For example, some runners find that they typically perform better in a hard workout after completing an easy run the preceding day than they do after a day of total rest. If this is the case for you, then you should probably schedule easy recovery runs between key workouts and take days off only when you really need them.

9. Long-Term Goal

Most runners—at least most runners under the age of 40—have at least one long-term goal. This is a performance goal that you wish to achieve eventually, but which requires more than a year's worth of additional development time, such that it cannot function as a short-term goal. Nevertheless, long-term goals can and should have an important bearing on your immediate training. There are various ways you can tweak the training you do in your next training cycle to put your development on the proper track toward your long-term goal (or goals) without affecting your ability to achieve your short-term goal.

Almost all of the runners I coach come to me fresh out of college, having never raced farther than 10 kilometers, and have long-term aspirations at the marathon distance. Most of them wait at least two years after college before attempting their first marathon, and I encourage them not to expect to run their lifetime-best marathon for another four to 10 years after that. During those transitional years, I prescribe training that will set up my runners for a successful marathon debut in a couple of years even as they continue to train for peak performance in races at the half-marathon distance and below. Specifically, they do more and longer long runs and long threshold runs than they would do if they never intended to run a marathon. This is one basic example of how a long-term goal can affect immediate training.

The other thing your long-term goals should do is encourage patience. As I explained in the above section on running experience, it takes years of consistent training to reach a level of development at which you are capable of performing the training that is necessary to achieve your lifetime-best race performances. If you understand this fact, you can mentally sketch out years of increasing and evolving training designed to develop your fitness step by step toward its lifetime-peak level, much as you plan out 12 to 24 weeks of increasing and evolving training to elevate your fitness step by step toward a short-term peak level within each training cycle. This little exercise should help you avoid rushing your development and training too hard and too soon. Your long-term planning does not require any detail, although it shouldn't take too much thought to settle on a general idea of the sort of training you will eventually have to do to achieve a specific long-term goal.

10. Motivational Profile

Individual runners are as different in their psychological makeup as they are in their physical characteristics. Certain psychological characteristics—which I lump together under the classification of "motivational profile"—have implications for how each runner should train that are as important as those physical characteristics. However, it's harder to formulate concrete guidelines for these psychological implications.

The gist of the matter is that each runner has certain motivational quirks that cause him or her to make training mistakes. It's important to understand what these quirks are and account for them in the planning (and execution) process as much as possible. Some quirks are motivational weak spots that must be addressed with measures that provide a motivational boost. Other quirks are motivational excesses that must be addressed with measures that apply a prudent braking force.

For example, some of the runners I coach have an excess of motivation that makes them feel compelled to "beat" the target pace times and split times I give them for workouts. In some workouts—specifically, in those that call for a maximal or near-maximal effort—this is not a problem, but in other workouts it is a problem. Running too fast in race-pace workouts is undesirable because the whole point of these workouts is to maximize race-pace-specific adaptations. I deal with my overeager runners by sometimes giving them target pace levels and split times that are slightly slower than I really want them to run, or by turning their hyper-competitiveness to their advantage by turning certain workouts into a pacing game, where the goal is to see how close they can come to "nailing" their targets perfectly. It might be a little harder for you to play such tricks on yourself than it is for me to play them on my runners, but if you have this compulsion to "better" your target times in every workout, you should give it a try.

One of the more common motivational weaknesses is a tendency to lose focus in one's training when there are long lapses between competitive opportunities. If you have this problem, you may need to schedule more frequent tune-up races than other runners do.

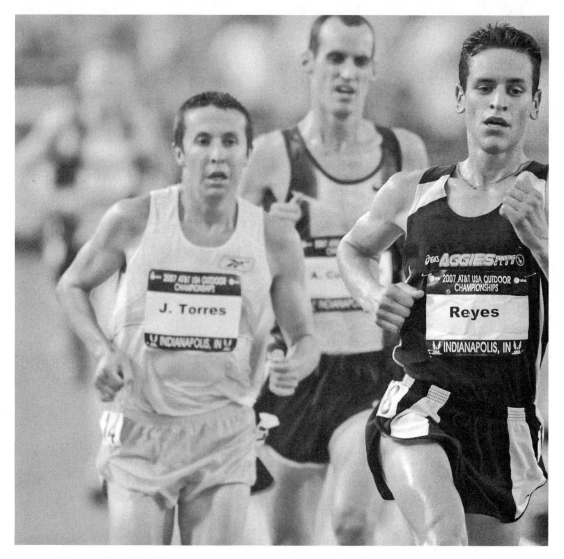

Jorge Torres © Alison Wade

Runner Profile: Jorge Torres

Jorge Torres and his twin brother, Edwardo, joined my team after graduating from the University of Colorado, where they ran for four years under the tutelage of coach Mark Wetmore. I've known Mark for more than 30 years, and I know his training philosophy intimately. He puts a strong emphasis on aerobic training, which is appropriate at the college level, so I could safely assume that Jorge had a strong aerobic foundation in place when he started working with me.

Jorge's long-term goal was to become a marathon runner, which meant that I needed to continue building his aerobic foundation with harder long runs, longer tempo runs, and more volume. At the same time, Jorge is naturally fast—he has a lot of fast-twitch muscle for a distance runner—and he had not yet done a lot of strength training at the time he began working with me. So I integrated more specific-endurance work and short intervals into his training as well. I was confident that this training emphasis would improve his performance at shorter distances, which would ultimately improve his performance in the marathon.

The risk I took with Jorge was that I basically gave him more of everything, and he had a history of frequent injuries and illnesses, so I knew I had to be careful with him. Fortunately, I discovered that in addition to being exceptionally fast, Jorge is also an exceptionally fast adapter, meaning his fitness level responds very quickly to new training challenges. This knowledge has enabled me to coax his fitness along slowly and carefully at most times and then get him race-ready very quickly with just a few hard sharpening workouts.

So far, so good. Jorge won the U.S. National Track and Field Championships at 10,000 meters in 2006 and is on track for a successful marathon debut at the time of this writing.

Creating a Training Plan

7

Creating your own training plan can be an intimidating prospect if you've never done it before. And the prospect of creating your own training plan based o n my adaptive running system—which is still rather new to you—might be even more intimidating. But rest assured that with a modest effort you can create your own, customized adaptive running training plan that will give you better race results than any ready-made plan you might choose to rely on.

Also, bear in mind that in the adaptive running system, training plans carry only limited responsibility for developing your race-specific fitness. Equally important is the process of choosing the most appropriate workout to do day by day (whether it's the workout in your plan, or a slightly different workout, or a totally different workout) based on your body's response to completed training. So even if the training plan you design isn't perfect (and no plan ever is), you can continually improve it on the fly.

The last chapter of this book presents a selection of ready-made adaptive running training plans. There's a low-volume, a moderate-volume, and a high-volume plan for each of the four popular road-race distances. You're welcome to choose and follow the most appropriate plan from this selection as a way to become more comfortable with the adaptive running system before graduating to creating your own training plan from scratch. To get the most out of these ready-made plans, you'll still have to modify workouts as you go based on your body's response to the workouts you've done. In doing so, you'll develop greater decision-making confidence and self-knowledge, which will help you design a better training plan when it's time to pursue your next peak-race performance.

You may also use the ready-made training plans in Chapter 12 as templates to guide you through the process of creating your own training plan. In the preceding chapters, I've given you a large number of tips and guidelines regarding how to develop your aerobic support, your neuromuscular fitness, and your specific endurance, but you have not yet seen how these three threads of training are woven together to create the fabric of a complete adaptive running training plan. The most important function of the plans in Chapter 12 is to provide this big picture. Each plan represents a standard adaptive running program that is customized only on the basis of peak-race distance and average running volume. You can use the plan that best suits you as a foundation for a more fully customized plan, which you'll create by making modifications based on the self-assessment guidelines provided in the previous chapter and the training-plan design guidelines presented in this chapter.

Or you can go straight to designing your own fully customized adaptive running training plan from scratch. This process has eight steps. They are as follows:

Step 1: Choose a peak race and a race goal.

Step 2: Pick a start date and plan duration.

Step 3: Decide on the appropriate running volume and frequency and weekly workout structure.

Step 4: Divide your plan into introductory, fundamental, and sharpening periods.

Step 5: Plan your peak training week.

Step 6: Schedule tune-up races and recovery weeks.

Step 7: Schedule progressions for interval workouts, threshold workouts, and long runs.

Step 8: Fill in the remainder of the schedule.

Let's now discuss each of these eight steps in detail. To make this discussion more concrete, I'll create an actual adaptive running training plan for a hypothetical runner as we go along.

Step 1: Choose a Peak Race and a Race Goal.

When it comes to designing training plans, the starting point is the endpoint. And the endpoint is a specific race in a certain place on a definite date. You may wish to do more than one race in the near future, but you will choose one as your top-priority peak race—the race you wish to start with peak fitness and finish with the best time you can possibly achieve. Until and unless you have chosen a peak race and a race goal to aim for, you don't even need a training plan. The whole purpose of designing a training plan is to create a sensible map of workouts leading from your current fitness state to a state of maximal race-specific fitness just in time for your peak race.

Choosing a peak race is something you can do with almost total freedom, as long as you exercise common sense, which, in my experience, most runners have. Common sense tells you not to choose a marathon taking place three weeks from now as your peak race if you've never run farther than 10 miles. Beyond this caution to exercise your best judgment, I am not here to tell you what your peak race should be. The purpose of choosing a peak race is to get yourself excited and to generate the motivation and focus you'll need to take your running to the next level. Only you can decide which peak-race option gets you most excited.

In most cases, you'll want to establish a time goal to achieve in your peak race. Running is primarily a sport of competition against oneself, and the stopwatch is the means by which we keep score in that competition. Setting ambitious but achievable time goals serves to increase one's motivation to train hard and give one's best effort in the race itself, and it often enhances the satisfaction of the race experience. Ultimately it matters little whether the goal is achieved. In fact, I'm fond of saying that the best goal setters achieve their race time goals only half the time. If you *always* achieve your race time goals, you are surely setting them too low. And if you *never* achieve your goals, clearly they are too ambitious.

How do you know what is an appropriate race time goal? As I mentioned in the previous chapter, if you have relevant past racing experience, then experience will guide you. Otherwise, just set a "guess goal" based on past performances at other race distances, on workout performances, or on how your fitness compares to that of training partners with experience at your peak-race distance. You'll be able to refine this goal as the training process unfolds and your peak race draws near.

For the purpose of illustrating the eight-step process of training plan design, let's choose a marathon peak race and a goal time of 2:39.

Step 2: Pick a Start Date and Plan Duration.

Another limitation on appropriate peak-race selection that I hinted at in the previous section is that the peak race must be far enough in the future to afford you enough time to train for optimal performance. On the other hand, it also should not be too far in the future or else you won't feel that all-important sense of urgency that motivates you to train hard, and you'll be at risk of peaking too early and becoming "stale" by race day. You may, however, choose a peak race that's many months in the future and simply delay the start date of formal training for that event until an appropriate time while focusing on other, more immediate goals.

The ideal duration of a training plan depends on the distance of the peak race and on your current fitness level. For most runners, longer races require more preparation time than shorter races because it takes a while to build the endurance needed to go the distance comfortably. The higher your current fitness level is, however, the less time you need to prepare for a race of any distance. The elite runners on my team maintain such a high fitness level throughout the year that they may devote only eight to 10 weeks of formal preparation to the marathon. In essence, they always have a solid foundation of introductory and early-fundamental-period training in their legs. Thus, at most times of the year their training is focused toward simply maintaining health and well-rounded fitness and inching their fitness in the direction of specificity to their next major competition. Only relatively short time blocks need to be devoted to aggressive, specific fundamental training and sharpening.

The situation of professional runners is unique in that they typically train to peak for three to four championship races per year. Thus, they are required to sketch out a plan for the entire year and to view the process of training for each championship race only semi-independently of the process of training for the others. The situation is very different for the typical amateur competitive runner, who aims for peak fitness only once or twice per year and does not sustain a consistently high level of fitness throughout the year, due to the other life priorities that periodically take time away from training, and to the occasional injury. (Elite runners get injured, too, but they are much more likely to maintain a high level of fitness despite their breakdowns thanks to aggressive rehabilitation and cross-training efforts.) Consequently, the type of training plan that is most often appropriate for the typical competitive runner is one that assumes a modest level of starting fitness and is strictly focused on a single peak race.

This is not to say that amateur competitive runners cannot design and follow yearlong, multi-peak training plans as most elite runners do. In fact, as an amateur competitive runner you stand to benefit no less than elite runners do from maintaining a consistently high level of fitness year-round and taking advantage of this fitness by peaking three or four times a year. Nevertheless, this approach just isn't realistic for most amateur competitive runners.

So, how long should your training plan be if you're in the typical situation of starting a training cycle at a level of fitness that is well below your desired peak fitness level? Simply put: Long enough to develop your fitness from its current level to the desired peak level at a rate that is neither hurried nor dawdling. In most cases, the optimal duration falls within the ranges presented in the following table.

Peak-Race Distance	Optimal Training-Plan Duration
5K	12–16 weeks
10K	14–18 weeks
Half-Marathon	16–20 weeks
Marathon	18–24 weeks

The higher your current fitness level is, the shorter your plan may be within the optimal range. The durations of the ready-made training plans presented in chapter 12 are 12 weeks for 5K, 14 weeks for 10K, 16 weeks for the half-marathon, and 20 weeks for the marathon. We will design a 20-week marathon training plan for the purpose of illustrating the training-plan design process.

Step 3: Decide on the Appropriate Running Volume and Frequency and Weekly Workout Structure.

Weekly running mileage is the most important variable that distinguishes individual training plans for the same peak-race distance. The best marathon training plan for one runner might have a peak volume of 40 miles in a week, while for another runner the peak running volume might be 120 miles in a week. If the runner for whom the 40-miles-per-week plan was most appropriate attempted to follow the 120-miles-per-week plan, she would quickly get injured. On the other hand, if the runner for whom the 120-miles-per-week plan was most appropriate followed the 40-miles-per-week plan, he would arrive at race day far short of peak fitness and fail to achieve his race goal.

To choose an appropriate peak weekly mileage target, consider your recent past training volume, how many times per week you plan to run, and the approximate distance you plan to run in your longest run. I recommend that every runner, including beginners, run at least six times per week, if possible. You need to exercise daily just for the sake of your health, and since you're a runner you might as well run every day. At the peak level of training, the typical weekday run should be at least four miles long. The peak length of the Sunday long run should be at least five miles for beginning 5K runners and 20 miles for beginning marathon runners. These parameters establish 25 miles as the lowest recommended peak weekly running volume level for beginning and very low-key competitive runners training for a 5K, and 40 miles for beginning and very low-key competitive runners training for a marathon.

The absolute bare minimum running frequency for progress as a runner is three times per week. If, for whatever reason, you choose to run only three to five times each week, I still recommend that you *work out* at least six times per week, doing some form of cross-training on your non-running days. If you've never run daily before, or have not done so in a while, you should not start doing so abruptly. The tissues of your lower extremities will need more than 24 hours to repair themselves and grow stronger between runs. Start with three or four short runs per week and do non-impact cross-training workouts on non-running days. After a few weeks, substitute a cross-training workout with a run and continue in this fashion until you're running six times per week.

Seventy miles is the maximum number of weekly miles you should attempt to pack into a training week that does not include more than one run per day on any day. If you're an experienced and highly competitive runner who is serious about achieving maximal performance but unwilling or unable to run twice on some days, then you should aim for a peak running volume of close to 70 miles per week, regardless of your peak-race distance.

For most experienced runners, running volume is limited by a lack of willingness to run more than a certain amount, given other life priorities, and not by an inability to run more. I cannot object to this choice. However, as a coach I am all too aware that the more you run, within your personal limits (which increase with training experience), the better you will perform. So my advice is that you gradually increase your running volume from one training cycle to the next until you reach the highest level you are comfortable with (in relation to a particular peak-race distance), and then hold it at that level. Avoid increasing your peak weekly running mileage by more than 50 percent compared to your most recently completed training cycle.

In chapter 3, I presented a table of weekly running mileage guidelines for five different categories of runner and for each of the four popular road-race distances. Use this table, the 50 percent rule, and the other guidelines given in this section to settle on an appropriate peak weekly running mileage for your next training plan. Like everything about adaptive running, this decision is subject to revision. You can scale your training volume up or back based on how your body responds to the workouts that you plan. Also, after completing the plan you can assess your general response to the volume level of the plan and use this assessment to settle on the best volume level for your next plan. For example, if you feel that the volume level was close to the maximal amount you could handle, but that your maximum increased slightly as an effect of experiencing the training process, you might choose to add 10 percent more running volume to your next plan.

To return to our illustration, let's suppose that our 20-week marathon training plan is being designed for a very competitive runner who has run as much as 60 miles a week and wants to improve on the race results he achieved through this level of training, but is unwilling to run more than once a day. Therefore we will set his maximal weekly running volume at 70 miles.

The final task to perform before you begin to schedule actual workouts is to establish a standard weekly workout schedule. Settling on a running frequency is a part of this task but not the whole of it—the other part is deciding which types of runs you wish to do on each day of the typical week. In my adaptive running system, it is standard to perform steep hill sprints (preceded by an easy run) on Monday, high-intensity runs (threshold runs, interval workouts) on Tuesday and Friday, and a long run on Sunday. I have found that this distribution of workouts provides the optimal balance of stress and recovery for the vast majority of runners. Thus, I recommend that you follow this template unless you have a compelling reason not to. If you do use this template, all you have to do is fill out the typical training week with the appropriate number of additional easy and moderate workouts. Following are suggested templates for 5, 6, 7, 10, and 12 runs per week.

5 Runs per Week (appropriate for 20–50 miles per week)						
Sunday	Monday	Tuesday	Wednesday	Thursday	Friday	Saturday
Long Run	Easy Run + Hill Sprints	Hard Run	Easy/ Moderate Run	Off or X-Train	Hard Run	Off or X-Train

6 Runs per Week (appropriate for 30–60 miles per week)						
Sunday	Monday	Tuesday	Wednesday	Thursday	Friday	Saturday
Long Run	Easy Run + Hill Sprints	Hard Run	Moderate Run	Easy Run	Hard Run	Off or X-Train

7 Runs per Week (appropriate for 45–70 miles per week)						
Sunday	Monday	Tuesday	Wednesday	Thursday	Friday	Saturday
Long Run	Easy Run + Hill Sprints	Hard Run	Moderate Run	Easy Run	Hard Run	Easy Run

10 Runs per Week (appropriate for 60–100 miles per week)						
Sunday	Monday	Tuesday	Wednesday	Thursday	Friday	Saturday
Long Run	AM: Easy Run + Hill Sprints PM: Easy Run	Hard Run	AM: Moderate Run PM: Easy Run	Easy Run	Hard Run	AM: Easy Run PM: Easy Run

12 Runs per Week (appropriate for 80–120 miles per week)						
Sunday	Monday	Tuesday	Wednesday	Thursday	Friday	Saturday
Long Run	AM: Easy Run + Hill Sprints PM: Easy Run	Hard Run	AM: Moderate Run PM: Easy Run	AM: Easy Run PM: Easy Run	AM: Hard Run PM: Easy Run	AM: Easy Run PM: Easy Run

Not every week in your training plan will be typical. In the first few weeks of training, you may need to ramp up to the running frequency that you will then sustain through the remainder of the training cycle. In planned recovery weeks, which should occur once every three or four weeks, you may do one or two runs fewer than you do in your typical week. And, of course, you will cancel, change, and shuffle workouts as necessary as you progress through the training plan.

Our hypothetical marathon runner will follow the seven-runs-per-week schedule presented above, except in the initial weeks of training and scheduled recovery weeks, when he will run six times a week.

Step 4: Divide Your Plan into Introductory, Fundamental, and Sharpening Periods.

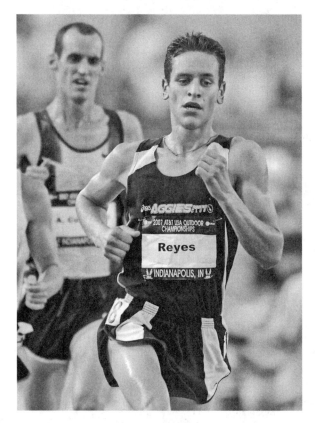

Before you make any other decisions about your training plan, decide how much and how often you will run. © Alison Wade

Training phases, or periods, as I call them, are not as sharply delineated in my adaptive running system as they are in other training systems, but I do not forego their use entirely. There is a natural sequence of short-term training priorities that punctuate the process of developing peak fitness, so it's natural to divide the training cycle into three relatively distinct periods, each focused on one of these priorities.

The first priority is developing an initial foundation of aerobic fitness and neuromuscular fitness that enables you to perform the more challenging training of the later periods effectively and without getting injured. The introductory period focuses on this priority. The second training priority is to build ever more race-specific fitness atop the twin foundation of basic aerobic fitness and neuromuscular fitness established in the introductory period. The fundamental period focuses on this second priority. The third and final training priority is to achieve peak-level race-specific fitness with a handful of very challenging race-specific workouts and rest up for your peak race. The sharpening period focuses on this last training priority.

The absolute and relative duration of each training period should be based on your starting fitness level, the distance of your peak race, and the total duration of your training plan. The higher your initial fitness level, the shorter your peak race, and the shorter your training plan, the shorter the introductory period may be. A mere two weeks of introductory training may suffice for an already fit runner starting a 12-week program culminating in a 5K peak race. If your starting fitness level is well below your peak fitness level, your introductory period should be longer—up to six weeks. Runners training for longer races are most likely to start at an initial fitness level that is far below their desired peak level, so the optimal introductory-period duration is almost always in the four-to-six-week range when the peak race is a half-marathon or a marathon.

The sharpening period should be four weeks long in almost every training plan. Two to three of these four weeks are devoted to putting the final edge on your race-specific fitness; the final one to two weeks comprise a tapering period. No runner requires or can handle more than a few weeks of true peak-level training, and no runner requires more than two weeks of reduced-volume training to rest up for a peak race.

The fundamental period is usually the longest training period because it must achieve the most movement in a runner's fitness. I recommend that you devote at least six weeks to fundamental training when preparing for a 5K or 10K peak race, and at least eight weeks when training for a half-marathon or marathon. In the training plans presented in chapter 12, the training-period breakdowns are loosely as follows:

	Duration of Phase (in Weeks)		
Peak Race	Introductory	Fundamental	Sharpening
5K	3	6	3
10K	4	6	4
Half-Marathon	6	6	4
Marathon	6	10	4

Our hypothetical marathon runner will use the same period breakdown as the marathon training plans in chapter 12. He is starting from a modest level of fitness. His training has been consistent, but lacking in challenging workouts and far below the volume level he will need to reach in the late fundamental period to achieve his race goal. Therefore a 20-week plan including a longer, six-week introductory period is appropriate.

Step 5: Plan Your Peak Training Week.

When you make a long car trip, you need to know the address of your final destination before you can decide whether you should turn left or right at the end of your driveway.

Likewise, when you are designing a training plan, you need to plan your peak week of training—the hardest week of training that immediately precedes your pre-race taper—before you can schedule appropriate training for the first week of the plan, the second week, and so forth. Your peak week can be either the week before your race week or two weeks before your race week. And by "peak week" I mean the week with your hardest race-specific workouts, not necessarily your highest mileage week.

Your peak week of training should feature three highly race-specific workouts: a set of specific-endurance intervals or a race-specific threshold workout on Tuesday, a race-specific threshold workout or a set of specific-endurance intervals on Friday, and some type of race-specific aerobic-support workout—a longer threshold workout or a faster long run—on Sunday. Schedule the usual easy run plus short hill sprints on Monday. The rest of the week is filler: easy and moderate runs whose number and duration fit the frequency and volume parameters you have set for your training plan.

The specific format for the three key workouts in your peak week of training will be determined by the distance of your peak race, your race goal, your volume level (the higher your overall training volume, the longer your peak workouts can be), and the guidelines for aerobic training, muscle training, and specific-endurance training presented in chapters 3 through 5.

Don't worry about planning the perfect workouts for the peak training week. As long as they closely simulate the challenges you will face in your peak race in slightly different ways, your peak workouts will do their job. In any case, like all other workouts, these workouts are planned in pencil. You may and probably will revise them at the 11th hour based on the state of your body entering your peak training week.

Following are examples of peak training weeks for runners training for four different race distances at four different mileage levels. All distances have been rounded to the nearest mile. The last example applies to our hypothetical 70-miles-per-week marathon runner for whom we are designing a complete, 20-week training plan.

5K Peak Training Week—30 Miles

Sunday	6 miles moderate 2-mile hard progression @ 10K pace
Monday	2 miles easy + 6 × 10-sec. steep hill sprint
Tuesday	1-mile warm-up 5 × 1K @ 5K pace with 90-sec. jog recoveries 1-mile cool-down
Wednesday	5 miles easy
Thursday	Off
Friday	1-mile warm-up 4 miles @ 10K pace 1-mile cool-down
Saturday	5 miles easy

10K Peak Training Week—80 Miles

	Workout 1	Workout 2
Sunday	2-mile warm-up 3 miles @ half-marathon pace 2 miles easy 3 miles @ half-marathon pace 2-mile cool-down	5 miles easy
Monday	5 miles easy + 10 × 10-sec. steep hill sprint	5 miles easy
Tuesday	2-mile warm-up 4 × 2K @ 10K pace + 1K maximum effort with 1-minute jog recoveries 2-mile cool-down	5 miles easy
Wednesday	5 miles easy + 2-mile moderate progression	5 miles easy
Thursday	5 miles easy	
Friday	1-mile warm-up 6 × 1 mile starting @ half-marathon pace, increasing to 10K pace 1-mile cool-down	5 miles easy
Saturday	8 miles easy + 2-mile hard progression	

Half-Marathon Peak Training Week—45 Miles

Sunday	12 miles moderate 2-mile hard progression @ half-marathon pace
Monday	6 miles easy + 8 × 10-sec. steep hill sprint
Tuesday	1.5-mile warm-up 4 × 2K @ 10K pace with 90-sec. jog recoveries 1.5-mile cool-down

Half-Marathon Peak Training Week—45 Miles	
Wednesday	6 miles easy + 2-mile hard progression
Thursday	Off
Friday	1.5-mile warm-up 4 × 3K @ half-marathon pace with 90-sec. jog recoveries 1.5-mile cool-down
Saturday	7 miles easy

Marathon Peak Training Week—70 Miles	
Sunday	10 miles moderate 10 miles @ marathon pace (6:00/mile)
Monday	6 miles easy + 10 × 10-sec. steep hill sprint
Tuesday	1.5-mile warm-up 4 × 3K @ half-marathon pace with 90-sec. jog recoveries 1.5-mile cool-down
Wednesday	8 miles easy + 2-mile hard progression (5:30/mile)
Thursday	6 miles easy
Friday	1-mile warm-up 3 miles @ half-marathon pace (5:45/mile) 1 mile easy 1 mile @ marathon pace 3 miles @ half-marathon pace 1-mile cool-down
Saturday	7 miles easy

Step 6: Schedule Tune-up Races and Recovery Weeks.

After planning your peak training week, you'll want to incorporate two non-workout elements into your training plan before you plot out the majority of your workouts. Those two elements are tune-up races and recovery weeks. It's sensible to tackle them at the same time, because tune-up races should be surrounded on both sides by at least two days of easy training whenever possible, so that you're sufficiently rested to perform well in them.

A recovery week is a week of training in which the workload is moderately reduced from the level of preceding weeks. The overall structure of the weekly training cycle remains essentially unchanged. Recovery weeks generally feature the same number, sequence, and types of workouts as normal training weeks, but workouts are shortened to achieve a 20- to 30-percent reduction in mileage. Recovery weeks give the body an opportunity to fully adapt to recent training and to prepare for a more challenging level of training in subsequent weeks. Competitive runners who typically maintain a workload that's close to the limit of what their bodies can handle require a recovery week every third week throughout the training cycle. Runners who maintain a more easily managed workload relative to their personal limits may only need a recovery week every fourth week. Low-key, low-volume competitive runners typically don't need to schedule recovery weeks at all. Instead, they can just take a day off or replace a hard run with an easy run as necessary.

If you consider the planned average training workload of your training plan to be very near your limit, then schedule a 20- to 30-percent mileage reduction every third week throughout the training plan as a baseline. If your planned average training workload is more moderate but still high enough that you anticipate needing the occasional recovery week, then schedule a 20- to 30-percent mileage reduction every fourth week throughout the training plan.

I encourage every runner to do at least one tune-up race preceding his or her peak race. Tune-up races have several benefits. First of all, they serve as key workouts that stimulate fitness gains exceeding those you get from any regular workout. Tune-up races also provide opportunities to achieve goals at race distances other than that of your primary peak race. It's not at all uncommon for a runner to set a 5K PR while training for a 10K peak race, for example, or to set a half-marathon PR several weeks before running a marathon. Finally, tune-up races provide the best evidence of your current fitness level.

If you're starting at a modest level of fitness, try to get at least eight solid weeks of training into your legs before toeing the line in a tune-up race. Avoid racing too often, as well. If you're racing on two weekends of every month, you're missing two Sunday long runs every month and are probably too sore and fatigued to train effectively on two Mondays and Tuesdays of every month. Shorter races take the least out of you, so if you like to race often, do mostly 5K's. Also, the shorter your peak race is, the more racing you can get away with, as 5K and 10K tune-up races provide specific training for 5K and 10K peak races. But if your peak race is a marathon, you'll get more benefit from a Sunday long run than from a 5K or 10K tune-up race, except on special occasions.

As a general rule, tune-up races should be shorter or no longer than your peak race. One exception is that a 10K is an acceptable tune-up race for a 5K peak race. You can get away with racing a half-marathon as a tune-up for a peak 10K, but you'll most likely get more out of another 10K.

A second general rule to follow in planning tune-up races is to do shorter tune-up races before longer ones. Eight weeks into a marathon training program, you'll most likely not be in good enough shape to run a decent half-marathon, but you might run a very strong 10K. It's best to save the half-marathon until roughly four weeks before your marathon.

Don't go out of your way to pick tune-up races that just happen to fall at the end of the recovery weeks you've scheduled for every third or fourth week throughout your training plan. Just schedule the tune-up races that make sense and adjust your recovery-week schedule as necessary. For example, suppose you normally take a recovery week every third week and you schedule a particular tune-up race that falls on the second Sunday after the preceding recovery week. In this case, it would make sense to train normally through Wednesday of that tune-up race week. Move Friday's key workout to Thursday and possibly scale it back a bit. Then run easy on Friday and run easy again or rest on Saturday. The following week, swap Tuesday's hard run with Wednesday's easy run so you have two solid recovery days after the tune-up race as well.

The following table shows a sensible schedule of tune-up races for training plans matching the durations of those presented in chapter 12. Our hypothetical marathon runner will follow the marathon tune-up race schedule shown here.

Peak Race:	5K	10K	Half-Marathon	Marathon
Plan Duration:	12 weeks	14 weeks	16 weeks	20 weeks
Tune-Up Races:	5K, Week 9	5K, Week 8 10K, Week 11	5K, Week 8 10K, Week 12	5K, Week 8 10K, Week 12 Half-marathon, Week 16

Step 7: Schedule Progressions for Interval Workouts, Threshold Workouts, and Long Runs.

The three "key workouts" that you do each week throughout an adaptive running training cycle—typically, but not always, an interval workout, a threshold run, and a long run—are the skeleton of your training plan. They provide the structure that your fitness development hangs on. Your other workouts merely "flesh out" the plan, so to speak.

In a standard adaptive running training schedule, your key workouts will fall on Tuesday, Friday, and Sunday. Your Tuesday and Friday workouts will focus on developing specific endurance from a foundation of aerobic support and neuromuscular fitness, primarily through intervals and threshold training, while your Sunday workout will usually be some type of long run. In chapters 3 through 5, I provided guidelines that you can use to plan standard key-workout progressions that are appropriate for each of the four popular road-race distances. The ready-made training plans in chapter 12 provide examples of standard key-workout progressions that are appropriate to different training volumes at each of those four distances. Chapter 6 provided guidelines that you can use to customize your key-workout progressions in ways that deviate from the standard, as necessary.

Use all of this information to create key-workout progressions for your entire training plan. To the degree that you feel unsure about how to proceed, stick close to the key-workout progressions in the ready-made training plan in chapter 12 that is most appropriate to the plan you're designing for yourself. But again, it's not important that each key workout be perfect in itself. As long as your three weekly key workouts evolve generally in the direction of those you'll do in your peak training week, you'll do fine. And again, you can always modify individual key workouts as necessary as the plan unfolds.

The following table presents a complete 20-week progression of key workouts for our illustrative marathon runner.

Week	Sunday	Tuesday	Friday
		Introductory Period	
1	8-mile easy run	6-mile easy run	6-mile easy run
2	10-mile easy run	6-mile easy run with 6 × 30-sec. fartlek intervals @ 10K–3K pace	5-mile easy run + 10-min. progression @ half-marathon pace (uphill, if possible)
3	12-mile easy run	6-mile easy run with 8 × 30-sec. fartlek intervals @ 10K–3K pace	6-mile easy run + 10-min. progression @ half-marathon pace (uphill, if possible)
4	8-mile easy run + 1.5 miles uphill @ goal marathon pace	7-mile easy run with 8 × 40-sec. fartlek intervals @ 10K–3K pace	5-mile easy run + 1.5-mile progression @ half-marathon pace (uphill, if possible)

Week	Sunday	Tuesday	Friday
Introductory Period			
5	9-mile easy run + 2 miles uphill @ goal marathon pace	7-mile easy run with 10 × 45-sec. fartlek intervals @ 10K–3K pace	5-mile easy run + 3-mile progression @ half-marathon pace (uphill, if possible)
6	9-mile easy run	6-mile easy run with 6 × 30-sec. fartlek intervals @ 10K–3K pace	5-mile easy run + 1.5-mile progression @ half-marathon pace (uphill, if possible)
Fundamental Period			
7	12 miles easy + 15 min. @ goal marathon pace	1.5-mile warm-up 6 × 800m @ 5K pace w/400m jog recoveries 1.5-mile cool-down	1.5-mile warm-up 2 × 1.5 miles @ 10K pace w/1-mile jog recovery 1.5-mile cool-down
8	5K tune-up race	1.5-mile warm-up 2 × (1 mile, 1K, 800m, 400m w/200m jog recoveries) @ 10K–1,500m pace 1.5-mile cool-down (on Wednesday)	1.5-mile warm-up 2 × 2 miles @ 10K pace w/1-mile jog recovery 1.5-mile cool-down
9	10 miles easy + 3 min. @ goal marathon pace	1.5-mile warm-up 6 × 800m @ 5K pace w/400m jog recoveries 1.5-mile cool down	1.5-mile warm-up 2 × 1 mile @ 10K pace w/1-mile jog recovery 1.5-mile cool-down
10	14 miles easy + 2 miles @ goal marathon pace	1.5-mile warm-up 5 × 1K @ 5K pace w/400m jog recoveries 1.5-mile cool down	1.5-mile warm-up 2 × 2.5 miles @ 10K pace w/1-mile jog recovery 1.5-mile cool-down
11	3 miles easy + 3 miles @ goal marathon pace	1.5-mile warm-up 5 × 1 mile @ 10K pace w/400m jog recoveries 1.5-mile cool-down	1.5-mile warm-up 3 miles @ half-marathon pace 1 mile easy 2 miles @ 10K pace 1.5-mile cool-down
12	10K tune-up race	1.5-mile warm-up 3 miles @ 10K pace 1.5-mile cool-down (on Wednesday)	1.5-mile warm-up 2 miles @ half-marathon pace 1 mile easy 2 miles @ 10K pace 1.5-mile cool-down
13	14 miles easy + 2.5 miles @ goal marathon pace	1.5-mile warm-up 3 × (1 mile, 1K, 800m, 400m w/200m jog recoveries) @ 10K–1,500m pace 1.5-mile cool-down	1.5-mile warm-up 4 miles @ half-marathon pace 1 mile easy 2 miles @ 10K pace 1.5-mile cool-down

Week	Sunday	Tuesday	Friday
		Fundamental Period	
14	5 miles easy + 5 × (1 mile @ marathon pace − 15 sec. per mile, 1 mile @ marathon pace + 1 min. per mile)	1.5-mile warm-up 4 × 2K @ 10K pace + 1K @ 5K–3K pace 1.5-mile warm-up 5 × 1 mile @ 10K pace w/400m jog recoveries 1.5-mile cool-down	1.5-mile warm-up 3 miles @ half-marathon pace 1 mile easy 3 miles @ 10K pace 1.5-mile cool-down
15	13 miles easy + 1.5 miles @ goal marathon pace	5 × 1 mile @ 10K pace	1.5-mile warm-up 4 miles @ half-marathon pace 1.5-mile cool-down
16	Half-marathon tune-up race	1.5-mile warm-up 3 miles @ marathon pace 1 mile easy 2 miles @ half-marathon pace 1 mile easy 1 mile @ 10K pace 1.5-mile cool-down (on Wednesday)	1.5-mile warm-up 2 × 3 miles @ half-marathon pace w/1-mile jog recoveries 1.5-mile cool-down
		Sharpening Period	
17	6 miles easy + 4 × (2 miles @ marathon pace − 5 sec. per mile, 1 mile @ marathon pace + 30 sec. per mile)	1.5-mile warm-up 4 × 3K @ half-marathon pace w/2-min. jog recoveries 1.5-mile cool-down	1.5-mile warm-up 4 × 2 miles @ half-marathon pace w/2-min. jog recoveries 1.5-mile cool-down
18	10 miles moderate 10 miles @ marathon pace (6:00/mile)	1.5-mile warm-up 4 × 3K @ half-marathon pace w/90-sec. jog recoveries 1.5-mile cool-down	1.5-mile warm-up 5 miles @ half-marathon pace 1.5-mile cool-down
19	17 miles easy	1.5-mile warm-up 3 × 3K @ half-marathon pace w/300m jog recoveries 1.5-mile cool-down	1-mile warm-up 3 miles @ half-marathon pace 1 mile easy 1 mile @ marathon pace 3 miles @ half-marathon pace 1-mile cool-down
20	12 miles easy + 3 miles @ goal marathon pace	1.5-mile warm-up 2 × 3K @ half-marathon pace w/300m jog recoveries 1.5-mile cool-down	1-mile warm-up 1 mile @ marathon pace 1 mile @ half-marathon pace 1-mile cool-down

Step 8: Fill in the Remainder of the Schedule.

The final step of the training-plan design process is to fill in the remainder of your training schedule with easy runs, moderate runs, steep hill sprints, strides, and drills. The volume of "filler" running should increase sensibly in the introductory period, starting at a level you can comfortably manage and building at a manageable rate toward the level you will sustain fairly consistently throughout the fundamental period.

In a standard adaptive running plan, steep hill sprints are introduced very cautiously (just one sprint per session) twice per week in week 2. Add one to two sprints per session per week until you reach the maximal level you're comfortable with and then cut back to one session per week. Replace the eliminated hill-sprint session with strides. Also, do strides and drills as part of your warm-up prior to any workout involving efforts at 10K pace or faster.

As you execute your training plan, just run the distance that feels right whenever an easy run is scheduled. The purpose of plotting specific distance numbers for easy and moderate runs in your training plan is not to lock yourself into running exactly the scheduled number of miles in each of them but rather to control your total weekly running volume appropriately.

Here is the complete, filled-in 20-week marathon-training plan for our invented runner.

20-Week Marathon Training Plan

Average Run Frequency: 7 days

Peak Volume: 70 miles/week

Introductory Period

Week 1	
Sunday	8 miles easy
Monday	Off
Tuesday	6 miles easy
Wednesday	5 miles easy
Thursday	5 miles easy
Friday	6 miles easy
Saturday	5 miles easy
Total miles: 35	

Week 2	
Sunday	10 miles easy
Monday	4 miles easy + 1 × 8-sec. hill sprint
Tuesday	6 miles easy w/6 × 30-sec. fartlek intervals @ 10K–3K pace
Wednesday	5 miles easy + 1-mile moderate progression
Thursday	4 miles easy + 1 × 8-sec. hill sprint
Friday	5 miles easy + 10-min. progression @ half-marathon pace (uphill, if possible)
Saturday	6 miles easy
Total miles: 42	

Week 3	
Sunday	12 miles easy
Monday	5 miles easy + 2 × 8-sec. hill sprint
Tuesday	6 miles easy w/8 × 30-sec. fartlek intervals @ 10K–3K pace
Wednesday	5 miles easy + 1-mile moderate progression
Thursday	5 miles easy + 2 × 8-sec. hill sprint
Friday	6 miles easy + 10-min. progression @ half-marathon pace (uphill, if possible)
Saturday	6 miles easy
Total miles: 48	

Week 4	
Sunday	8 miles easy + 1.5 miles uphill @ goal marathon pace
Monday	6 miles easy + 4 × 8-sec. hill sprint
Tuesday	7 miles easy w/8 × 40-sec. fartlek intervals @ 10K–3K pace
Wednesday	7 miles easy + 1-mile moderate progression
Thursday	5 miles easy + 4 × 8-sec. hill sprint
Friday	6 miles easy + 1.5-mile progression @ half-marathon pace (uphill, if possible)
Saturday	6 miles easy
Total miles: 49	

Week 5	
Sunday	9 miles easy + 2 miles uphill @ goal marathon pace
Monday	6 miles easy + 5 × 10-sec. hill sprint
Tuesday	7 miles easy w/10 × 45-sec. fartlek intervals @ 10K–3K pace
Wednesday	7 miles easy + 1-mile moderate progression
Thursday	5 miles easy + 5 × 10-sec. hill sprint
Friday	5 miles easy + 3-mile progression @ half-marathon pace (uphill, if possible)
Saturday	8 miles easy
Total miles: 53	

Week 6 (Recovery Week)	
Sunday	9 miles easy
Monday	Off
Tuesday	6 miles easy w/6 × 30-sec. fartlek intervals @ 10K–3K pace
Wednesday	7 miles easy + 1-mile moderate progression
Thursday	6 miles easy + 4 × 10-sec. hill sprint
Friday	6 miles easy + 1.5-mile progression @ half-marathon pace (uphill, if possible)
Saturday	6 miles easy
Total miles: 43	

Fundamental Period

Week 7	
Sunday	12 miles easy + 2 miles @ goal marathon pace
Monday	6 miles easy + 6 × 10-sec. hill sprint
Tuesday	1.5-mile warm-up 6 × 800m @ 5K pace w/400m jog recoveries 1.5-mile cool-down
Wednesday	6 miles easy + 2-mile moderate progression
Thursday	6 miles easy + drills and strides
Friday	1.5-mile warm-up 2 × 1.5 miles @ 10K pace w/1-mile jog recovery 1.5-mile cool-down
Saturday	8 miles easy
Total miles: 57	

Week 8	
Sunday	5K tune-up race (2-mile warm-up, 1-mile cool-down)
Monday	6 miles easy + 6 × 10-sec. hill sprint
Tuesday	7 miles easy + 2-mile moderate progression
Wednesday	1.5-mile warm-up 2 × (1 mile, 1K, 800m, 400m w/200m jog recoveries) @ 10K–1,500m pace 1.5-mile cool-down
Thursday	6 miles easy + drills and strides
Friday	1.5-mile warm-up 2 × 2 miles @ 10K pace w/1-mile jog recovery 1.5-mile cool-down
Saturday	8 miles easy
Total miles: 52	

Week 9 (Recovery Week)	
Sunday	10 miles easy + 3 min. @ goal marathon pace
Monday	Off
Tuesday	1.5-mile warm-up 6 × 800m @ 5K pace w/400m jog recoveries 1.5-mile cool down
Wednesday	6 miles easy + 6 × 10-sec. hill sprint
Thursday	6 miles easy + drills and strides
Friday	1.5-mile warm-up 2 × 1 mile @ 10K pace w/1-mile jog recovery 1.5-mile cool-down
Saturday	6 miles easy
Total miles: 42	

Week 10	
Sunday	14 miles easy + 2 miles @ goal marathon pace
Monday	6 miles easy + 6 × 10-sec. hill sprint
Tuesday	1.5-mile warm-up 5 × 1K @ 5K pace w/400m jog recoveries 1.5-mile cool down
Wednesday	6 miles easy + 2-mile moderate progression
Thursday	6 miles easy + drills and strides
Friday	1.5-mile warm-up 2 × 2.5 miles @ 10K pace w/1-mile jog recovery 1.5-mile cool-down
Saturday	10 miles easy
Total miles: 63	

Week 11	
Sunday	13 miles easy + 3 miles @ goal marathon pace
Monday	6 miles easy + 6 × 10-sec. hill sprint
Tuesday	1.5-mile warm-up 5 × 1 mile @ 10K pace w/400m jog recoveries 1.5-mile cool-down
Wednesday	6 miles easy + 2-mile hard progression
Thursday	6 miles easy + drills and strides
Friday	1.5-mile warm-up 3 miles @ half-marathon pace 1 mile easy 2 miles @ 10K pace 1.5-mile cool-down
Saturday	10 miles easy
Total miles: 65	

Week 12 (Recovery Week)	
Sunday	2-mile warm-up 10K tune-up race 1-mile cool-down
Monday	Off
Tuesday	6 miles easy + 6 × 10-sec. hill sprint
Wednesday	1.5-mile warm-up 3 miles @ 10K pace 1.5-mile cool-down
Thursday	6 miles easy + drills and strides
Friday	1.5-mile warm-up 2 miles @ half-marathon pace 1 mile easy 2 miles @ 10K pace 1.5-mile cool-down
Saturday	8 miles easy
Total miles: 44	

Week 13	
Sunday	14 miles easy + 2.5 miles @ goal marathon pace
Monday	6 miles easy + 6 × 10-sec. hill sprint
Tuesday	1.5-mile warm-up 3 × (1 mile, 1K, 800m, 400m w/200m jog recoveries) @ 10K–1,500m pace 1.5-mile cool-down
Wednesday	6 miles easy + 2-mile moderate progression
Thursday	6 miles easy + drills and strides
Friday	1.5-mile warm-up 4 miles @ half-marathon pace 1 mile easy 2 miles @ 10K pace 1.5-mile cool-down
Saturday	8 miles easy
Total miles: 66	

Week 14	
Sunday	5 miles easy + 5 × (1 mile @ marathon pace − 15 sec. per mile, 1 mile @ marathon pace + 1 min. per mile)
Monday	6 miles easy + 6 × 10-sec. hill sprint
Tuesday	1.5-mile warm-up 4 × 2K @ 10K pace + 1K @ 5K–3K pace 1.5-mile cool-down
Wednesday	6 miles easy + 2-mile hard progression
Thursday	6 miles easy + drills and strides

Week 14	
Friday	1.5-mile warm-up 3 miles @ half-marathon pace 1 mile easy 3 miles @ 10K pace 1.5-mile cool-down
Saturday	10 miles easy
Total miles: 66	

Week 15 (Recovery Week)	
Sunday	13 miles easy + 1.5 miles @ goal marathon pace
Monday	6 miles easy + 6 × 10-sec. hill sprint
Tuesday	1.5-mile warm-up 5 × 1 mile @ 10K pace w/400m jog recoveries 1.5-mile cool-down
Wednesday	6 miles easy + 2-mile hard progression
Thursday	6 miles easy + drills and strides
Friday	1.5-mile warm-up 4 miles @ half-marathon pace 1.5-mile cool-down
Saturday	8 miles easy
Total miles: 59	

Week 16	
Sunday	1.5-mile warm-up Half-marathon tune-up race 1-mile cool-down
Monday	6 miles easy + 6 × 10-sec. hill sprint
Tuesday	6 miles easy + 2-mile hard progression
Wednesday	1.5-mile warm-up 3 miles @ marathon pace 1 mile easy 2 miles @ half-marathon pace 1 mile easy 1 mile @ 10K pace 1.5-mile cool-down
Thursday	6 miles easy + drills and strides
Friday	1.5-mile warm-up 2 × 3 miles @ half-marathon pace w/1-mile jog recovery 1.5-mile cool-down
Saturday	11 miles easy
Total miles: 68	

Sharpening Period

Week 17	
Sunday	8 miles easy + 4 × (2 miles @ marathon pace − 5 sec. per mile, 1 mile @ marathon pace + 30 sec. per mile)
Monday	6 miles easy + 6 × 10-sec. hill sprint
Tuesday	1.5-mile warm-up 4 × 3K @ half-marathon pace w/2-min. jog recoveries 1.5-mile cool-down
Wednesday	6 miles easy + 2-mile hard progression
Thursday	6 miles easy + drills and strides
Friday	1.5-mile warm-up 4 × 2 miles @ half-marathon pace w/400m jog recoveries 1.5-mile cool-down
Saturday	7 miles easy
Total miles: 71	

Week 18	
Sunday	10 miles moderate 10 miles @ marathon pace (6:00/mile)
Monday	6 miles easy + 6 × 10-sec. hill sprint
Tuesday	1.5-mile warm-up 4 × 3K @ half-marathon pace w/300m jog recoveries 1.5-mile cool-down
Wednesday	6 miles easy + 3-mile moderate progression
Thursday	6 miles easy + drills and strides
Friday	1.5-mile warm-up 2 × 3 miles @ half-marathon pace w/1-mile jog recovery 1.5-mile cool-down
Saturday	8 miles easy
Total miles: 71	

Week 19 (Taper Week)	
Sunday	17 miles easy
Monday	Off
Tuesday	1.5-mile warm-up 3 × 3K @ half-marathon pace w/300m jog recoveries 1.5-mile cool-down
Wednesday	5 miles easy + 1-mile moderate progression
Thursday	4 miles easy + drills and strides

Week 19 (Taper Week)	
Friday	1-mile warm-up 3 miles @ half-marathon pace (5:45/mile) 1 mile easy 1 mile @ marathon pace 3 miles @ half-marathon pace 1-mile cool-down
Saturday	4 miles easy
Total miles: 50	

Week 20 (Taper Week)	
Sunday	12 miles easy + 3 miles @ goal marathon pace
Monday	Off
Tuesday	1.5-mile warm-up 2 × 3K @ half-marathon pace w/300m jog recovery 1.5-mile cool-down
Wednesday	4 miles easy + 1-mile hard progression
Thursday	4 miles easy
Friday	1-mile warm-up 1 mile @ marathon pace 1 mile @ half-marathon pace 1-mile cool-down
Saturday	2 miles easy
Total miles: 37	
Sunday	Marathon goal race in 2:39

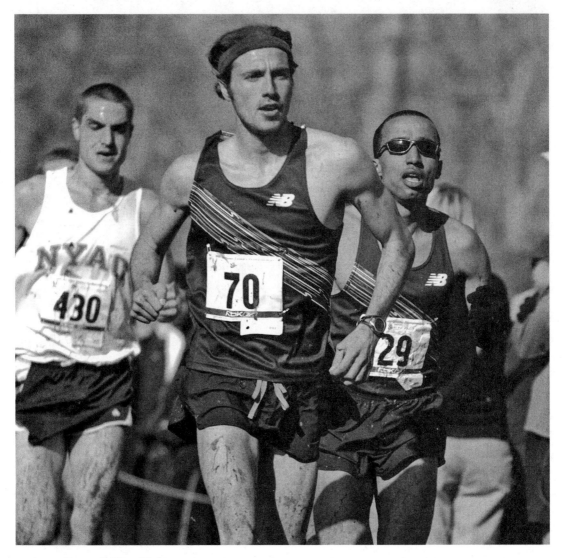

James Carney © Alison Wade

Runner Profile: James Carney

My work with James Carney exemplifies how adjusting your training for a better custom fit can lead to rapid improvement in racing, even if you're already an experienced and highly trained runner. James was indeed experienced and highly trained when he joined my team in the winter of 2007. He was 26 years old with four years of experience on an elite running team coached by Bob Sevene in California and four years of college running experience before that. His personal best times of 13:47 for 5,000 meters and 28:27 for 10,000 meters were slower than those of the other male runners on my team, but I felt he had the potential to improve substantially.

I had no idea just how quickly he would improve, however. James responded extremely well to the new training approach he experienced with me. His past training was more conventional in certain ways, with long blocks of training that focused on just one or two types of training, and especially long blocks of mostly moderate-intensity aerobic work. My adaptive running system emphasizes diverse and varied workouts throughout the training process, and that's exactly what James got when he moved to Boulder. I introduced challenging threshold work into his regimen at the very beginning, as well as steep hill sprints, which he had never done before. In addition, I increased the amount of specific-endurance training in his program while slightly reducing his volume of aerobic work, because he had already developed a strong aerobic system.

James's first race as part of my team was the 2007 USA National Cross-Country Championships, held only nine weeks after I gave him his first adaptive running workout. He had a breakthrough performance, finishing seventh, qualifying for the World Championships, and defeating several big-name runners he had never even come close to beating before. Two months later, James achieved an even greater breakthrough, lowering his 10,000-meter personal best to 27:43 and establishing himself among the first rank of American runners.

Few experiences have done more to boost my confidence that I am a pretty good coach than my first few months of working with James Carney.

Training Execution

8

One of the best ways to ensure that your next training cycle ends in disaster is to stubbornly endeavor to complete every workout in your training plan exactly as designed, no matter what. In the most likely scenario, early in the training process you'll develop a sore spot in your knee, shin, or elsewhere that becomes more and more painful because you refuse to heed the warning and you continue doing all of your scheduled workouts. After another week or two, the sore spot will have developed into a full-blown overuse injury that renders you completely unable to continue training.

In the only other likely scenario, sooner or later you will push through a hard workout that's scheduled on a day when you happen to be unexpectedly fatigued from previous training, and as a result, instead of making you stronger, the workout will thrust you deeper into a hole of fatigue that leaves you in an even worse state when it comes time to do your next hard workout. After another week or two of persisting in this manner, you'll find yourself feeling exhausted in every single workout, and perhaps even between workouts. Your fitness will plateau and then begin a downward spiral, despite (or rather, due to) the fact that your training workload continues to increase. In a matter of time you will wind up sick or injured and completely unable to continue training.

A training plan is just that: a plan. It is not a set of laws, commandments, or marching orders that you must live and die by and never deviate from. Your training plan represents an ideal scenario: the sequence of workouts that you hope to be able to perform if everything goes as expected. But things do not always go as expected in the execution of a training plan. Somewhere along the journey you are certain to experience at least one and probably many more than one period of poor recovery or substandard performance, a trouble spot in your body, an illness or nutrition-related problem, or an unanticipated course of development such as lagging neuromuscular fitness or signs that you are approaching a fitness peak too early. When such things happen, you must depart from the course of workouts laid out in your training plan to stay on course toward your peak-race goal.

Within the past year, I've had to make such adjustments in the training of every athlete I coach. In the early spring, Dathan Ritzenhein developed a stress reaction in his foot while performing a speed workout on the track. Dathan has a history of stress fractures, so I took aggressive action and had him cease all land running and instead do all of his workouts on an anti-gravity treadmill that enabled him to run on as little as 65 percent of his body weight, pain-free. When he returned to land running, we found that he had lost very little fitness, so we picked up his preparations for the summer track season right where we had left off, but pushed back his first race by a couple of weeks.

Also within the past year, middle-distance runner Jo Ankier of Great Britain overtrained over the winter and became run-down. Her workout and race performances slipped, and she just felt generally lousy. I responded by adding more rest and recovery days to her schedule, removing much of the "filler" from her training, and concentrating her hard work in just a couple of workouts each week. She rebounded quickly and was racing well again by April.

I could give you other examples involving Ed Torres, Jason Hartmann, and my other athletes, but I trust my point has been made. It pays to train responsively, modifying your planned training in small ways or big ways as necessary, based on what happens over the course of the training process. Many competitive runners resist such deviations, either because they assume that to give up on planned training is to give up on achieving their peak-race goal, or because they simply don't know how to stray from the course of their planned training to stay on course toward their goal. Making training adjustments on the fly is easier for runners who have a coach they trust. Self-coached runners like you must develop the openness and knowledge to steer your own training in response to what happens as the process unfolds.

To achieve your best performance in a peak race, two things are required: a solid training plan and successful training execution. Successful training execution is a matter of deviating from your plan in appropriate ways as necessary from the first day of training to the last. This doesn't mean that your training plan goes out the window the moment you put it into action. To the contrary, as you proceed through the training cycle, you will complete each and every workout as prescribed in your training plan unless you have a good reason to do otherwise.

Good reasons to deviate from scheduled workouts range from residual fatigue and soreness from previous workouts to feeling that your body requires or will benefit more from a different sort of training stimulus than the one that the prescribed workout would provide. Relying on your training plan without over-relying on it in this manner will give you the best chance of running to your full potential in your peak race.

There are three levels of training adjustments that you must be open to and confident in making to get the best results from a training cycle: single-workout adjustments, multi-workout adjustments, and adjustments affecting the remainder of a training cycle.

Single-Workout Adjustments

The first requirement for successful training execution is listening to your body every day. Listening to your body means paying attention to how your body feels during and between workouts and adjusting your running accordingly. Plan A is always to do your originally scheduled workouts, of course, but you should always be ready and willing to move to plan B or C, if necessary, and in most cases you should not be at all worried when you do find it necessary to scrap today's plan A.

On days when you have a hard workout planned, scan your body for any signals that it's not prepared for the workout. If you feel especially fatigued and/or sore in the hours preceding a planned hard workout, consider replacing it with an easier workout or, in extreme cases, taking the day off. It's often difficult, however, to accurately predict how you'll feel and perform during a workout based on how you feel in the hours preceding it. Therefore I recommend that, except in those cases where you're certain that you need to cancel or modify a planned hard workout, you at least start the planned workout regardless of how you feel and then simply cut it short if you find that you feel lousy and are unable to perform adequately.

The only factor that I have found to be a reasonably accurate predictor of readiness for a hard workout 24 hours later is performance in steep hill sprints. That's one reason my standard adaptive running training week places them on Mondays and sometimes also on Thursdays—in each case, one day before a hard threshold or interval workout. If you lack power and feel drained and flat when performing a set of hill sprints, it is at least somewhat likely that you will perform poorly in any type of hard workout you try to do the following day. The reason hill sprints are an especially good indicator of readiness for hard training is that they place a high demand on the neuromuscular system and thereby reveal underlying nervous-system fatigue that you might not notice otherwise.

An Australian study found that a five-jump broad-jump test was a very reliable indicator of inability to perform at normal levels in a 3K running time trial for a group of triathletes subjected to a period of especially hard training. A five-jump broad-jump test challenges the neuromuscular system in a way that is similar to the way steep hill sprints do. I have found that hill sprints are not equally reliable as a recovery-status indicator for all runners, however, so pay attention to how you tend to perform in hard workouts undertaken the day after a substandard hill-sprint session before you begin using them to make anticipatory training adjustments.

Unless you get sick or develop an outright injury, always try to get at least a small training stimulus of the special kinds called for each day in the standard adaptive running training week (or your custom-modified version thereof). Here, once more, is the basic adaptive running weekly template for special training stimuli:

Sunday	Monday	Tuesday	Wednesday	Thursday	Friday	Saturday
Long Run	Steep Hill Sprints	Intervals or Threshold Training			Intervals or Threshold Training	

Plan A, again, is always to perform the exact session that you scheduled for yourself when designing your training plan. Plan B, when you feel lousy, is to perform a shortened version of the same session. For example, instead of 30 minutes of threshold running you might do only 15 minutes and call it a day. Typically, this approach is better than postponing a planned workout until the next day, because then you may have to postpone the next planned hard workout, and so forth. In other words, there's a domino effect. So when your body tells you that it isn't prepared to handle even a shortened version of a planned hard workout, go ahead and cancel it (plan C) instead of postponing it and hope to feel stronger when it's time for your next hard workout.

Up to this point, we've talked about replacing planned hard training with easier training or rest when you feel unexpectedly bad. But does it also work the other way? Should you replace easy runs with hard workouts when you feel unexpectedly strong? Generally, I do not advise that you spontaneously replace planned easy runs with hard workouts on those days when you feel especially strong. Just enjoy the feeling and perhaps add a short, fast progression (say, 10 minutes of "hard" running) onto the end of the run to indulge your body's urge to pour on the gas. By conserving your strength in this manner, you'll increase the chances that you feel strong again when it comes time to do your next hard workout, when running hard and well will provide more benefit.

It's okay to make the occasional exception to this rule when you're confident that it's the right move. For example, suppose you're training for a marathon. Tomorrow you have a 12-mile long run with a 1-mile moderate progression scheduled. Last week you did a 10-mile long run with a 1-mile progression and you felt surprisingly strong at the end. Normally you increase the distance of your long runs very gradually, because past experience has taught you that your endurance builds slowly. But you have a feeling that you now have an opportunity to be a little more aggressive—that you could handle a 13-miler with a 1.5-mile progression tomorrow. Even if you return to a more conservative long-run build-up in subsequent weeks, taking advantage of this opportunity will put your endurance development slightly ahead of schedule, so you decide to give it a try. You can always make the decision to return to plan A during the workout if you don't feel as strong as you expected.

In most cases, however, when you feel especially strong in a planned hard workout, the proper way to take advantage of the situation is not to lengthen the workout but simply to run a little faster than normal. But in doing this, stay true to the intended intensity level(s) called for. If, for example, a workout calls for 5K of threshold running at your current 10K pace, don't turn the workout into a 5K time trial just because you feel great. Instead, take pleasure in the discovery that your current 10K pace is a bit faster than anticipated and run the 5K threshold segment at your true, revised current 10K race pace.

It doesn't pay to "get greedy" in your training. In a well-designed training plan, you'll have opportunities to run to the point of significant fatigue. It's best to save these efforts for their appointed times. If it should turn out that your entire training plan is unexpectedly easy, make your *next* training plan more challenging, but don't risk spoiling the current one by getting too aggressive.

Multi-Workout Adjustments

Another way of listening to your body that is critical to effective training execution involves continuously paying attention to how your body is adapting to your training throughout the cycle. The main objective of doing this is to assess whether your fitness development is on track and on schedule to reach the level of race-specific fitness that you'll need to attain your peak-race goal, and to determine precisely how you are off track or off schedule, if indeed you are. Typically, the discovery that your fitness development is off track requires that you adjust more than one scheduled workout.

In order to know whether your fitness is on track or off track, you must remain mindful of the final destination of your training, which is specific endurance for your peak-race goal; in other words, the capacity to cover the full peak-race distance at your goal pace. This destination is represented in the peak training week that you laid out when designing your training plan. You must be able to perform as expected in the highly challenging and race-specific workouts contained in this peak week of training to achieve your peak-race goal. So your peak training week is the nearest thing to an unchangeable, etched-in-stone decree in the whole adaptive running system. If you have to change it substantially, you probably have to change your goal. (I'll come back to this topic later in the chapter.)

The workouts that you scheduled for the weeks preceding your peak training

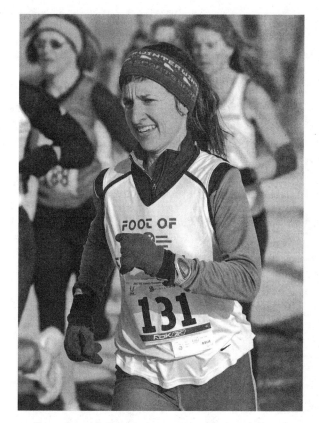

If your lungs feel strong but your legs feel weak in speed workouts, your neuromuscular fitness may be lagging. © Alison Wade

week represent the training progression that, based on your knowledge and experience, will do the best job of developing your fitness step by step from the level it's at when you start training to the desired peak level. As you execute the training plan, however, you'll inevitably find that you were slightly wrong—that your body doesn't respond to the training progression exactly as you had expected it to. Adjusting your planned workouts sensibly over the course of executing your training will increase the odds that you are able to complete your peak training week more or less as planned and achieve your peak-race goal.

There are essentially three ways in which your fitness can fail to measure up to the expectations you had when you designed your training plan. Your aerobic fitness, your neuromuscular fitness, or your specific endurance could lag too far behind the other two components of your running fitness. The following table provides a concise summary of signs that your fitness is possibly off track in one of these three ways.

Throughout the training process, closely monitor your fitness development by looking for the following signs that your neuromuscular fitness, your aerobic fitness, or your specific endurance might not be where it should be.

Table 8.1 Signs that Your Fitness Might Be Off Track	
Signs that your neuromuscular fitness is lagging	• You feel sluggish in your speed workouts • You fell weak when running uphill • In threshold runs, your breathing is under control but your legs feel heavy
Sign that your aerobic fitness is lagging	• You fatigue faster than you feel you should during long runs • You feel fast in speed-interval workouts, but you fatigue after just a few intervals • In threshold workouts, your legs seem to want to go faster than your lungs can handle
Signs that your specific endurance is lagging	• You have trouble sustaining your goal race pace in specific endurance workouts • You fatigue faster than you should in specific endurance workouts • You don't perform as well as expected in a spec test • You perform poorly in a tune-up race

Experiencing one of the signs identified in table 8.1 does not automatically indicate that your training is flawed and should be adjusted. You cannot expect to perform well in every workout, nor can you expect your neuromuscular fitness, aerobic fitness, and specific endurance to always be on the same level throughout the training process. For example, if you are naturally a speed runner, and your muscular system is stronger than your aerobic system, it will be normal for you to feel that your lungs rather than your legs are limiting your performance in threshold workouts. Presumably, if you are such a runner, you designed a training program that accounts for your strengths and weaknesses using the guidelines presented in chapter 6.

My purpose in encouraging you to watch out for signs of possible flaws in your fitness development is not to have you hit the proverbial panic button and overhaul your training every time you observe such a sign, like a bad investor who watches the stock market too closely and moves his money around too often instead of taking the long view. When monitoring your fitness development, you need to keep a sense of perspective that helps you brush off certain signs as nothing to worry about and react only to those signs that demand a response. Understanding the final destination of your training and keeping it always in mind will enable you to maintain the perspective needed to accurately judge whether your fitness is truly off track to the degree that requires a multi-workout adjustment.

This process is really a matter of developing and acting on hunches. It's impossible to formulate a strict set of rules to apply in the process of considering possible adjustments to planned workouts. You have to go by a sense of feel or intuition that is informed by your knowledge of adaptive running and of yourself as a runner. In any case, it's not something you need to worry too much about, because the training adjustments you'll make in response to this type of diagnosis are not drastic.

The guiding principle for multi-workout adjustments is simple: If your neuromuscular fitness is lagging, add more muscle training to your next two or three weeks of training, while possibly also slightly reducing your aerobic-support and/or specific-endurance training. If your aerobic fitness is lagging, add more aerobic-support training to your next two or three weeks of training, while possibly also slightly reducing your muscle and/or specific-endurance training. And if your specific endurance is lagging, add more specific-endurance training to your next two or three weeks of training, while possibly also slightly reducing your muscle and/or aerobic-support training. After executing your adjusted workouts, reassess your fitness balance and then decide whether to continue with this altered balance of training types or revert back to your training plan.

To give you a feeling for how to make these multi-workout adjustments, I'll present three sample scenarios. In scenario #1, a runner who's currently in the fundamental period of training for a 10K peak race decides that her neuromuscular fitness is lagging and adjusts her next three weeks of training to provide more muscle-training stimulus. In scenario #2, the same runner decides that her aerobic fitness is lagging and adjusts her next three weeks of training to provide more aerobic stimulus. And in scenario #3, the same runner decides that her specific endurance is lagging and adjusts her next three weeks of training to provide more specific-endurance stimulus. First I'll present the originally planned next three weeks of training. The three alternative scenarios then follow.

Planned Training

This three-week training progression represents the training that our hypothetical 10K runner had originally planned to do before an assessment of her fitness development led her to conclude that one component was lagging, necessitating a multi-workout adjustment.

Sunday	Monday	Tuesday	Wednesday	Thursday	Friday	Saturday
7 miles easy + 1-mile moderate uphill progression	4 miles easy + 6 × 10-sec. hill sprint	1-mile warm-up 2 × 2 miles @ half-marathon pace w/ 1-mile jog recovery 1-mile cool-down	4 miles easy	Off	1-mile warm-up 8 × 400m @ current 5K pace w/ 2-min. jog recoveries 1-mile cool-down	5 miles easy + 2 sets strides and drills
7 miles easy + 2-mile moderate progression	4 miles easy + 6 × 10-sec. hill sprint	1-mile warm-up 2 × 2.5 miles @ half-marathon pace w/ 1-mile jog recovery 1-mile cool-down	4 miles easy	Off	1-mile warm-up 8 × 600m @ current 5K pace w/ 2-min. jog recoveries 1-mile cool-down	5 miles easy + 2 sets strides and drills

Sunday	Monday	Tuesday	Wednesday	Thursday	Friday	Saturday
8 miles easy + 2-mile moderate progression	4 miles easy + 6 × 10-sec. hill sprint	1-mile warm-up 2 miles @ half-marathon pace 1 mile easy 2 miles @ 10K pace 1-mile cool-down	5 miles easy	Off	1-mile warm-up 8 × 800m @ current 10K–5K pace w/ 2-min. jog recoveries 1-mile cool-down	5 miles easy + 2 sets strides and drills

Scenario #1

In this scenario, the originally planned three-week training progression has been modified to provide slightly more muscle-training stimulus, based on the runner's assessment that her neuromuscular fitness is lagging. (Modified workouts appear in **boldface.**)

The extra muscle work has been added primarily to Tuesday's workouts, which were focused on threshold efforts in the original schedule. The amount of threshold work in these workouts has been reduced to "make room" for this muscle work and avoid overtraining. To compensate, Sunday's long-run progressions have been changed from moderate (normally a little faster than marathon pace) to hard (roughly half-marathon pace). This prevents the runner from losing momentum in the development of her aerobic support in the process of accelerating the development of her neuromuscular fitness.

Sunday	Monday	Tuesday	Wednesday	Thursday	Friday	Saturday
7 miles easy + **1-mile hard uphill progression**	4 miles easy + 6 × 10-sec. hill sprint	1-mile warm-up **3 miles @ half-marathon pace 4 × 300m hills @ 1,500m pace** 1-mile cool-down	4 miles easy	Off	1-mile warm-up 8 × 400m @ current 5K pace w/ 2-min. jog recoveries 1-mile cool-down	5 miles easy + **3 sets strides and drills**

Sunday	Monday	Tuesday	Wednesday	Thursday	Friday	Saturday
7 miles easy + **2-mile hard progression**	4 miles easy + 6 × 10-sec. hill sprint	1-mile warm-up **2 × (1 mile, 800m, 400m, 200m) @ 10K–1,500m pace, w/ 400m jog recoveries** 1-mile cool-down	4 miles easy	Off	1-mile warm-up 8 × 600m @ current 5K pace w/2-min. jog recoveries 1-mile cool-down	5 miles easy + **3 sets strides and drills**
8 miles easy + **2-mile hard progression**	4 miles easy + 6 × 10-sec. hill sprint	1-mile warm-up 2 miles @ half-marathon pace 1 mile easy 2 miles @ 10K pace 1-mile cool-down	5 miles easy	Off	1-mile warm-up 8 × 800m @ current 10K–5K pace w/2-min. jog recoveries 1-mile cool-down	5 miles easy + **3 sets strides and drills**

Scenario #2

In this scenario, the originally planned three-week training progression has been modified to provide slightly more aerobic-support training stimulus, based on the runner's assessment that her aerobic fitness is lagging. (Modified workouts appear in **boldface**.)

Only a very slight amount of volume is added to the schedule—to minimize the risk of overtraining—but it should suffice to measurably accelerate the runner's aerobic-support development nonetheless. Adding a mile or two to each Sunday long run will make these workouts more fatiguing, thereby stimulating greater aerobic adaptations. Adding progressively longer progressions to the end of Wednesday's easy runs will give the runner additional time at the upper end of her aerobic intensity zone. There is no need to reduce muscle training or specific-endurance training in this scenario.

Sunday	Monday	Tuesday	Wednesday	Thursday	Friday	Saturday
8 miles easy + 1-mile moderate uphill progression	4 miles easy + 6 × 10-sec. hill sprint	1-mile warm-up 2 × 2 miles @ half-marathon pace w/ 1-mile jog recovery 1-mile cool-down	4 miles easy **+ 1-mile moderate progression**	Off	1-mile warm-up 8 × 400m @ current 5K pace w/ 2-min. jog recoveries 1-mile cool-down	5 miles easy + 2 sets strides and drills
9 miles easy + 2-mile moderate progression	4 miles easy + 6 × 10-sec. hill sprint	1-mile warm-up 2 × 2.5 miles @ half-marathon pace w/1-mile jog recovery 1-mile cool-down	4 miles easy **+ 1.5-mile moderate progression**	Off	1-mile warm-up 8 × 600m @ current 5K pace w/ 2-min. jog recoveries 1-mile cool-down	5 miles easy + 2 sets strides and drills
10 miles easy + 2-mile moderate progression	4 miles easy + 6 × 10-sec. hill sprint	1-mile warm-up 2 miles @ half-marathon pace 1 mile easy 2 miles @ 10K pace 1-mile cool-down	**4 miles easy + 2-mile moderate progression**	Off	1-mile warm-up 8 × 800m @ current 10K–5K pace w/2-min. jog recoveries 1-mile cool-down	5 miles easy + 2 sets strides and drills

Scenario #3

In this scenario, the originally planned three-week training progression has been modified to provide slightly more specific-endurance training stimulus, based on the runner's assessment that her specific endurance is lagging. (Modified workouts appear in **boldface.**)

In the first week, the original threshold workout is replaced with a set of specific-endurance intervals. Sunday's long run is shortened and the progression is replaced with a threshold effort to compensate for the change in Tuesday's workout without increasing the week's overall training workload and thus risking overtraining. In the second week, the only change is to Sunday's run, in which the progression is replaced with a 1.5-mile race-specific effort performed in a prefatigued state. With a solid specific-endurance interval workout also scheduled for Friday, this one change is sufficient. In the third week, Sunday's long run is shortened and fartlek intervals at 10K pace are added to it. Tuesday's threshold workout is tweaked just a bit to make it a little more race-specific.

In this scenario, overall (aerobic) training volume is modestly scaled back to accommodate additional specific-endurance work. The result will be a boost in specific endurance without risk of overtraining or loss of neuromuscular or aerobic fitness.

Sunday	Monday	Tuesday	Wednesday	Thursday	Friday	Saturday
6 miles easy + 2 miles @ half-marathon pace	4 miles easy + 6 × 10-sec. hill sprint	1-mile warm-up **4 × 1 mile @ current 10K pace w/400m jog recoveries** 1-mile cool-down	4 miles easy	Off	1-mile warm-up 8 × 400m @ current 5K pace w/2-min. jog recoveries 1-mile cool-down	5 miles easy + 2 sets strides and drills
7 miles easy + 1.5 miles @ 10K pace	4 miles easy + 6 × 10-sec. hill sprint	1-mile warm-up 2 × 2.5 miles @ half-marathon pace w/ 1-mile jog recovery 1-mile cool-down	4 miles easy	Off	1-mile warm-up 8 × 600m @ current 5K pace w/2-min. jog recoveries 1-mile cool-down	5 miles easy + 2 sets strides and drills
9 miles easy with 8 × 1-min. fartlek intervals @ 10K pace scattered throughout	4 miles easy + 6 × 10-sec. hill sprint	1-mile warm-up **2 × 2 miles @ goal 10K pace with 1-mile jog recovery** 1-mile cool-down	5 miles easy	Off	1-mile warm-up 8 × 800m @ current 10K–5K pace w/2-min. jog recoveries 1-mile cool-down	5 miles easy + 2 sets strides and drills

It is possible for two or three components of your running fitness to lag simultaneously. Such a general lag in fitness development is usually a sign that you are overtraining and requires a different sort of multi-workout adjustment. Specifically, it requires that you take a few easy days and/or rest days and then resume normal training at a slightly reduced workload compared to your original plan.

Adjustments Affecting the Remainder of a Training Cycle

Major setbacks such as injuries and illnesses may require adjustments that affect the remainder of the training cycle, and perhaps also your peak-race goal. In most cases, a typical overuse injury need not have a drastic effect on your training and peak-race goal. It is usually possible to prevent the injury from becoming serious by immediately ceasing to run as soon as pain raises a red flag and to maintain fitness by cross-training while the injury heals and then make a fairly smooth return to training after a few days, or a few weeks at most. But an illness such as a 10-day flu will render you unable to do any training whatsoever and will probably necessitate a slow and cautious return to training even after its symptoms have disappeared.

Anytime you miss more than five days of training due to illness or any other cause, adjust your future training in the following manner: In your first two or three days back on the roads, run by feel and run cautiously. Start at an easy pace and run only as long as you feel comfortable. If you feel good, speed up and run farther, but don't go overboard. On your third or fourth day back, perform a challenging specific-endurance workout to assess how much fitness you've lost. If you find that you've lost little fitness, then work toward resuming your normal training—not immediately, but gradually over the next 10 days or so. If you find that you've lost substantial fitness, scrap your original training plan and create a new one that takes your fitness from its present level to the highest level possible in the time available before your peak race. Also, create a new peak-race goal that is commensurate to the level of fitness you can reasonably expect to achieve in the time remaining.

Canceling a peak race is a difficult decision to make, but sometimes it's the right one. If the best peak-race performance you can hope to achieve after missing some training is so far below the level you had hoped to achieve that it just doesn't seem worth the effort, then it's probably not worth the effort. Find a new peak race to aim for that's at least a few weeks later and start a new training cycle to prepare for it.

Training Through Injuries

Professional runners have become much smarter about avoiding and overcoming injuries than they were in my days on the circuit. The professional runners of my generation tried too often to push through injuries, which usually resulted in making them worse. The only other alternative, it seemed to us, was to take time off and lose fitness voluntarily. Only a few smart runners aggressively pursued cross-training as a compromise between trying to continue running as normal despite injury pain and taking time off. Those who did were more often able to reach the starting line of important races in one piece and ready to perform at a high level. Since racing is a professional runner's livelihood, cross-training as a means of "salvaging" a training cycle affected by injury started to catch on. These days, most elite runners in the United States rely on cross-training to maintain fitness while an injury heals—and to prevent injuries from becoming severe in the first place.

The Dathan Ritzenhein example I shared at the beginning of the chapter is typical. The foot problem he experienced during his spring ramp-up for the summer track season easily could have ruined his racing plans had he tried to push through it, or even if he had responded to it by ceasing to exercise completely. But by immediately ceasing his land running and training just as hard on an anti-gravity treadmill for four weeks, Dathan was able to stay fit and heal, and as a result his foot injury turned out to be only a minor setback.

You probably don't have access to an anti-gravity treadmill, but you can train through injuries in more or less the same way using cross-training options such as bicycling, inline skating, and elliptical training. Whenever you experience pain in a bone, muscle, or joint that affects your running, immediately stop running and transfer your workouts to your preferred cross-training activity until you're able to run pain-free again. Try to keep the frequency, duration, and intensity of workouts the same in your cross-training activity as they would have been if you hadn't gotten injured and had continued to follow your training plan.

Resist any temptation to resume running before the injury has fully healed. When you're fairly confident that the injury has healed, do one or two more cross-training workouts for good measure and then do a test run. If this workout goes well, you may then return to following your training plan.

Most competitive runners do not particularly enjoy cross-training. Dathan nearly went insane with boredom when running as many as 130 miles a week on that space-age treadmill. But the surest way to minimize the time you have to spend cross-training instead of running (and the surest way to minimize the amount of time you are injured) is to react to pain experienced during running very quickly. The more readily you abandon your training plan by switching from running to cross-training when injury pain begins, the more closely you will be able to follow your original plan in the long run.

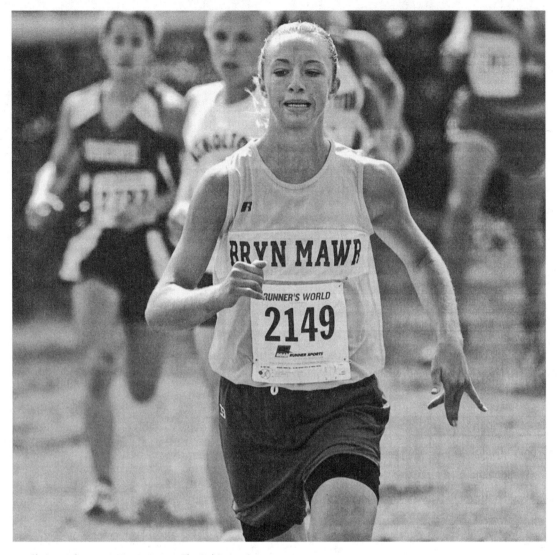

Christy Johnson © Kim Hairston, *The Baltimore Sun*

Runner Profile: Christy Johnson

Christy Johnson is one of the first runners I coached, and one of the only high school runners I have coached. Christy's parents approached me about their daughter as she was preparing for her junior year of competition. She had demonstrated considerable talent in her first two years of high school running, setting PRs of 2:23 for 800 meters and 5:30 for 1,600 meters, but her progress had been thwarted by frequent injuries, including stress fractures and knee pain. After explaining to Christy's parents what sort of approach I would use to keep their daughter healthy and guide her development, they decided I was the right man for the job and I worked with her for the next two years.

The training program Christy had followed in school lacked balance. It featured far too much specific work and not enough emphasis on muscle training and aerobic support. I corrected the problem by reducing Christy's specific work to one interval session and one fartlek run per typical week; giving her lots of steep hill sprints, which boosted her strength tremendously; and expanding her base of easy aerobic running.

Throughout my first year of coaching Christy, I had only one goal, which was to keep her healthy, knowing that, if I could achieve this goal, performance would follow. Keeping Christy healthy required that I be very flexible with her training—never looking too far ahead, paying close attention to how her body responded to workouts, and always trying to give her the workout she would benefit most from each day.

This approach worked very well. At the end of her junior year, Christy won the Colorado State Championship at 800 meters. Her family moved to Maryland for Christy's senior year, during which I continued advising her and she lowered her personal best times to 2:13 for 800 meters and 4:54 for 1,600 meters. Christy is now a top varsity runner at Princeton University.

Improving from Year to Year

9

If you take up the sport of distance running as a child, you can expect to continue improving until you're well over 30 years of age, and to remain at your performance peak until you're pushing 40. And regardless of how old you are when you start running, you can expect to be able to improve gradually for at least six or seven years. So if you start running at age 40, there's a pretty good chance you will be significantly faster when you're 47.

There's a difference, of course, between being able to improve over such a long period of time and actually doing so. Many runners who would love nothing more than to continue improving for many years hit a premature peak due to inconsistent training, injuries, failure to build properly on past training, failure to learn from experience, or even failure to believe in their ability to reach higher. Most runners who stop improving before they feel they should blame another factor: lack of time for the additional training that's needed for ongoing improvement; but this notion is a fallacy. I've never met a nonelite runner who was training so perfectly that he or she could only improve by training more.

Taking the long view is an important facet of adaptive running. After all, adaptation of any sort takes time, and to achieve any significant degree of adaptation, such as reaching one's genetic limit of physiological adaptation to running, usually takes a very long time. As a coach, my ultimate objective is not just to help my runners achieve their goal for the next race or the upcoming season; rather, it is to set each runner on a steady course of improvement and to keep him or her on that course of improvement as long as possible. Above all, I want my runners to race better this year than last year, and to race better next year than this year.

There are six keys to improving from year to year as a runner. I keep each of them constantly in mind when charting a course for the development of my athletes. The six keys are:

1. Consistency

2. Avoiding injuries

3. Building on past training

4. Learning from experience

5. Experimentation

6. Setting higher goals

Let's take a close look at each of them.

Consistency

When you stop running or reduce your training workload, the fitness adaptations that you worked so hard to achieve begin to reverse themselves. Exercise scientists refer to this process as "detraining." The rest of us refer to it as getting out of shape. Different aspects of detraining proceed at different rates, but most of them proceed all too quickly, producing an almost immediate and rapidly worsening decline in performance. For example, the concentration of aerobic enzymes in the muscles may begin to decline within two days after a runner stops training. A study from the early 1990s found that performance in a high-intensity treadmill running test decreased by more than 9 percent in a group of runners who stopped running cold-turkey for two weeks. Other research has shown that runners lose fitness when their training is interrupted at a significantly faster rate than they gain fitness when they ramp up their training.

It is very difficult to improve as a runner without consistency in your training. When a reduction or interruption in training causes you to lose fitness, you dig a hole for yourself that takes much longer to climb out of than it took to create. By contrast, when you maintain a solid foundation of fitness through consistent training, it is much easier to achieve a higher level of performance through modest short-term increases in training workload and/or improvements in training practices.

Lack of consistency in training is one of the most common barriers to improvement in nonelite competitive runners. Some training interruptions are caused by injuries, which I will discuss in the next section. But there is another common type of training lapse that is more easily avoided: off-season slacking. Many runners simply voluntarily get out of shape during the winter, when the weather is foul, the days are short, and there are no races on the horizon. Having lived, trained, and coached for many years in Boulder, Colorado, where the winters can be truly savage, I have empathy for those runners who slack in the off-season. I would even say that a certain amount of off-season slacking is acceptable and even healthy. Everyone needs a break now and then. But the unavoidable fact is that if you want to improve from year to year, you have to stay in decent shape through the winter.

It isn't too difficult to get a break from the physical and mental grind of race-focused training without losing much fitness. You can cross-train indoors (cycling, aerobics, etc.) or outdoors (snowshoeing, mountain biking, etc.) to keep your aerobic system sharp while at the same time escaping the pounding of running and enjoying the motivational boost that comes with variation. You may even enhance some aspects of your fitness—particularly your strength—by focusing on certain types of cross-training that you have less time for during the rest of the year. Calisthenics, weightlifting, and Pilates workouts are all good options. But whatever you do, don't go cold turkey on running. A week's break is fine, but otherwise you should try to run at least twice a week throughout the winter to maintain the adaptations to repetitive impact that only running provides and that take so long to regain once you've lost them.

If you are a longtime off-season slacker, I think you'll be amazed to discover how much easier it is to reach a higher level of performance in the spring if you maintain a solid foundation of fitness over the winter.

Avoiding Injuries

Injuries are the most common factor that thwarts training consistency at all levels of the sport of running. Improvement in running is very difficult to come by if you're frequently injured. But if you're able to stay healthy for an extended period of time and avoid other training interruptions, improvement becomes virtually automatic.

Over the years I've observed many cases of runners who achieved stunning levels of improvement simply by overcoming a pattern of bodily breakdowns and getting into a groove of steady training. A great example is Shalane Flanagan. A promising runner in her college and early professional years, Flanagan saw her career seriously derailed in 2005, at age 25, when she developed a major foot injury that required surgery and months of rehabilitation to fix. When she was finally able to return to normal training, Flanagan felt a renewed hunger to improve, and improve she did. In January 2007 she smashed her personal best time for 3,000 meters indoors by 21 seconds, clocking 8:33—a new American record. Three months later, she bettered her 5,000-meter PR by an equal amount, setting another new American record in the process. Flanagan's mid-career breakthrough shocked many people, including her, but the recipe was nothing new:

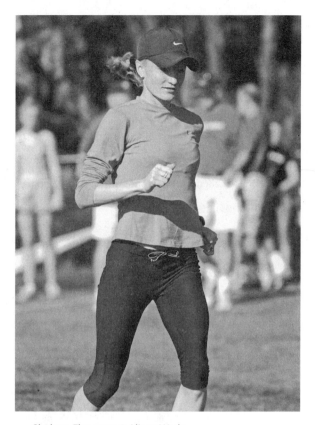

Shalane Flanagan © Alison Wade

Consistent, dedicated training unleashing potential previously hidden by injuries.

Preventing injuries is the most important priority of training. Injuries foil progress more than anything else, yet the harder you push for progress in your training, the more likely it is that you will get injured. Thus, if you don't prioritize injury prevention with specific practices, you're very likely to break down sooner or later.

The most effective way to prevent injuries is to avoid running in pain. Whenever unusual pain manifests in a bone, muscle, or joint, stop running and don't start running again until you can do so pain-free. The surest way to prevent pain from emerging in the first place is to never increase your training workload abruptly or do workouts that are substantially harder than any workout you've done recently. Maintaining a consistently high running workload will help you avoid making such dangerously sudden increases.

As I've mentioned more than once already, running steep hill sprints at least once a week drastically reduces injury susceptibility by significantly strengthening the muscles and joints. Traditional core-muscle training is a good supplement to hill sprints. Running with proper technique is also important. If you're a heel striker, learn to run flat-footed. This will reduce the risk of knee injuries and shin splints especially. Always wear the lightest, most comfortable running shoes you can find, and replace them every 500 miles. Finally, healthy eating plays a key role in injury prevention as well. Include a nice balance of food types (fruits, vegetables, meats, dairy, seafood, and whole grains) in your diet, minimize the amount of processed, sugary, and fried foods you consume, and make sure you get enough calories.

Building on Past Training

Each training cycle you complete changes your body. When you begin a new training cycle, you are not the same runner you were when you started the last one. Therefore, you should not train in precisely the same way that you did in your last training cycle, no matter how successful it was. In fact, in some ways, the more successful your last training cycle was, the more you can and should change the next one.

For example, suppose you struggled to handle the volume of running you planned for your last training cycle. If this is the case, the last thing you want to do is increase your training volume in the next training cycle. But you just might be able to handle the same running volume more comfortably in the next one, supposing you take a short break to rejuvenate your body and ease back into hard training. If, on the other hand, the running volume you planned for your last training cycle seemed ideal—enough to build your fitness to a high level but not so much that you struggled with it—then you'll probably be able to increase your running volume slightly in the next training cycle. The "summit" of your recently completed training cycle is now the foundation for the next.

Increasing your training volume is the simplest way to stimulate year-to-year improvement by building on past training, but it is not the only way, nor is it always the best way. At some point in their development, all runners reach a point where their training volume is either as high as they can take it without sacrificing the quality of their workouts, or as high as they care to take it given the need to balance running with other priorities in life. After this point is reached, the only way to build on past training is to increase the specificity of your training. And even before you reach your lifetime running-volume limit, increasing the amount of race-specific training you do from year to year is an important way to build on past training and stimulate further improvement.

Over the course of your running career, the arc of your training evolution should move from generality toward specificity, just as it does within each individual training cycle in the adaptive running system. When you start running, your training should place a heavy emphasis on aerobic development and muscle training—the twin foundations of running fitness. Your specific-endurance training should be limited; do just enough to sharpen up for races. In subsequent training cycles, build on your foundation by increasing your total running volume and by doing tougher aerobic workouts (longer and faster long runs and threshold runs) and more challenging muscle-training sessions.

When foundation-building has taken you about as far as it will take you, begin adding more and more specific-endurance work to your training—that is, more work in the 3K-to-half-marathon pace range. Each year, find a way to add slightly more of this type of training to your regimen, whether it is by introducing it earlier in the training cycle, by doing longer specific-endurance workouts, or by adding a little extra specific-endurance work into other workouts besides those that are entirely focused on specific endurance.

The movement from generality to specificity can only go so far, of course. Even the most seasoned runners can only handle so much specific-endurance training. Moderate aerobic-pace running will necessarily always account for the majority of your weekly miles, because your body can handle a lot of this type of training and because doing a lot of it gives you a foundation to handle more specific-endurance training. Your year-by-year increases in specific-endurance training should be quite modest and should cease as soon as you reach a point at which you feel you're doing as much specific-endurance running as your body will ever be able to handle.

Very few competitive runners really take advantage of this long-view approach to training evolution. By becoming one of the few who do, you will improve much more steadily and for a longer span of time than you would otherwise.

Learning from Experience

Perhaps the most important skill you can develop to foster improvement in your running is that of learning from experience. By that I mean paying attention to how your body responds to various training patterns, determining what works for you and what doesn't, and modifying your future training to include more of what does work and less of what doesn't. The most valuable service I provide the runners I coach is the application of this skill to their training. Cultivating the ability to learn from experience is the key to becoming an effective self-coach.

The reason that the ability to learn from experience is so important is that each runner is unique. If the same training methods worked equally well for every runner, there would be no need to pay attention to how your body responds to them. But because there's no predicting how your body will respond to individual workouts, let alone long-term training patterns, ongoing improvement depends on your ability to assess the effectiveness of workouts and training patterns and to make appropriate adjustments based on these assessments.

Day-by-day adjustments are needed to keep your training on track toward a particular race goal, but year-to-year improvement requires a broader scope of analysis. In November or December, after the year's last race is in the books, I sit down with each of my runners to comprehensively analyze the past season. We talk about what went right and what went wrong, and we try to identify the training patterns that seemed to do the most good and those that seemed to do more harm than good. Based on these discussions, we make some decisions about how we'll approach next year's training: what we'll do similarly and what we'll do differently.

You should do the same thing as a self-coached runner. During your off-season break, set aside some time to look at your training log and race results with a view toward identifying any specific lessons they might offer. A full year of training and racing is hardly a controlled experiment. There are so many variables at play that it's impossible to establish precise cause-and-effect relationships between particular training patterns and particular fitness results with perfect certainty. But if you have indeed paid close attention to your body over the course of the year and kept a good training log, your hunches will generally be fairly accurate. Following is a list of questions you might want to ask yourself during your year-end review, plus some ideas about how to use your answers in planning your approach to next year's training.

Did I perform as well as expected in my peak races?

The ultimate objective of your training is to maximize your performance in peak races. So your peak-race performances are the first things you should look at when assessing your past year's training. Every runner prefers a satisfying peak-race performance to a disappointing one, but the silver lining around disappointing peak-race performances is that they provide better learning opportunities.

Sometimes a disappointing peak-race performance results from unrealistic expectations, but this scenario is much more likely to affect inexperienced runners than experienced ones. Perhaps the most common cause of failure to meet realistic expectations in a peak race is peaking too early. Runners often spend too much time doing specific, high-level training before a peak race and consequently do their best running several weeks early. If you feel you were running better a month or so before a peak race than you did in the race itself, and you did in fact sustain high-level, race-specific training for some time before the race, then consider modifying next year's training in ways that will ensure that you don't peak early again. Specifically, concentrate your peak-level training closer to the actual peak race. Extend your fundamental period of training so that you've achieved a higher level of general fitness when you begin doing hard, specific work.

In other cases, a disappointing peak-race performance results from the opposite cause. You fail to peak at all because you don't allow enough time to build peak-level fitness and/or you don't do enough peak-level training before the race. If your training cycle leading up to a disappointing peak race was compressed or hurried, plan a longer training cycle next year. And if your training cycle did not culminate with at least four solid weeks of peak-level training featuring lots of challenging race-specific workouts, be sure that your next training plan includes a sharpening period that fits this description.

Another common cause of disappointing peak-race performance is failure to taper properly. Some runners race best when they engage in a modest taper, approaching the pre-race week as they would a normal recovery week. Other runners race best when they taper more drastically, starting their taper 10 days to two weeks before a peak race and reducing

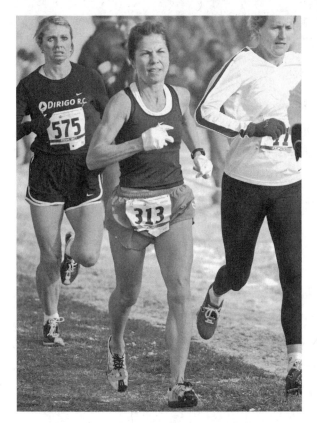

Sometimes a bad race is due to a bad taper, not necessarily bad training. © Alison Wade

their training to a minimal level in the final week. If you feel that a poor taper might be the cause of a disappointing peak race in the past year, consider trying a different sort of taper next year. If your taper was short and modest, try a longer and/or sharper taper. If your taper was fairly extreme, try doing a taper that's more like a normal recovery week.

How did I perform in my tune-up races?

After assessing last year's peak-race performances, assess your tune-up race performances. Runners often perform better in tune-up races than they do in peak races. This phenomenon may indicate that the runner peaked too early and should modify his or her future training to avoid a repetition of this scenario.

It's also common for runners to perform very poorly in tune-up races that fall early in the training cycle and to run steadily better in subsequent races. While this pattern does suggest that the runner's training was effective, it usually also indicates that the runner started the training cycle at a relatively low fitness level and that much of the training cycle was wasted on playing catch-up. As I suggested above, I believe it is important to sustain a high level of base fitness year-round, so that when you begin formal training for a peak race you don't have to play catch-up and can instead train in a way that builds on your solid foundation and takes your running performance to new heights.

If a tendency to get out of shape between training cycles is the probable explanation for poor performance in your early tune-up races, try to plan next year's training in a way that enables you to stay consistently fit and start each training cycle at a higher level.

Did my running volume hold me back in any way?

After assessing your race performances, next look back over your training logs and consider the volume of running you did over the past year. Estimate your average weekly running mileage, determine your peak weekly running mileage, and note the size of volume fluctuations throughout the year. Now try to establish a cause-and-effect relationship between these volume numbers and the fitness development and race results you achieved in the past year.

Ask yourself the following questions: Could my body have handled more mileage than I took on last year? If so, is it likely that running slightly more miles would have improved my fitness and performance? In other words, was I held back by inadequate running volume? Or did I try to run too much last year? Would I have performed better in my key workouts if I had run slightly less in other workouts? Was I frequently fatigued or injured due to excessive mileage?

In answering these questions, bear in mind that problems that seem to result from excessive training volume are often caused by excessive *fluctuations* in running mileage. Injuries and overtraining fatigue tend to develop during periods of increasing running volume. If you allow your running volume to fall too low at one or more times during a running season, you have to devote more time to the process of making relatively larger volume increases when you begin focused preparation for a peak race. As a result you're likelier to run more miles than your body is prepared to handle. If you experienced large fluctuations in your training volume last year, concentrate on making your running volume more consistent next year. If you do, you'll probably find that the peak running volume that seemed to be too much last year is easily handled and more productive this time around.

Was my training poorly balanced?

Most runners are also held back by the *quality* of running they do as much as they are by the *quantity* of running they do. Specifically, their training lacks balance. Every competitive road racer should consistently include the following training stimuli in his or her training: easy runs, long runs, threshold runs, specific-endurance intervals, speed intervals, and maximal efforts (e.g., short hill sprints). The majority of your weekly running should be done at lower intensities, and only a tiny fraction should be done at maximal intensity, but no training stimulus should ever be overemphasized or marginalized. Very few nonelite runners train with appropriate balance. Improving the balance of your training stimuli is a simple way to improve your running without training more, or even harder, necessarily.

Was I limited by my aerobic fitness?

A "performance limiter" is a relative weakness in your running fitness that is the primary factor preventing you from performing better at any given time. If your aerobic fitness is underdeveloped relative to your neuromuscular fitness and specific endurance, then aerobic fitness will be your limiter. If your neuromuscular fitness is lagging behind your aerobic fitness and specific endurance, then neuromuscular fitness will place a ceiling on your running performance. And if your specific endurance is weaker than your aerobic fitness and neuromuscular fitness, then your specific endurance will hinder your overall fitness development.

A sure way to improve your running next year is to analyze your past year of running, identify your primary limiter, and find ways to address it in next year's training. Start with aerobic fitness. There are several possible signs that you were limited by your aerobic fitness in the past year. The first is a tendency to perform better in shorter races than in longer races. Another sign of lagging aerobic fitness is a trend of stronger performance in shorter, faster workouts than in longer, slower workouts. Did you tend to feel substantially stronger running intervals at 1,500-meter to 3K pace than you did running threshold workouts at 10K to half-marathon pace? If so, then aerobic fitness was probably your Achilles' heel. Poor recovery between workouts may also indicate relatively low aerobic fitness.

There are three ways to address limiting aerobic fitness in planning next year's training. First, you can increase your overall running volume by adding one or more additional easy runs to your weekly schedule or by slightly increasing the average distance of your easy runs. This option is most appropriate for less experienced runners who have run low mileage in the past and feel ready and willing to run more. A second option is to increase the average intensity of your aerobic training by adding more threshold work to your schedule, tacking faster progressions onto the end of some easy runs, and incorporating faster running into your long runs. This is a good option for runners with at least a couple of years of training experience in their legs who are limited in their ability or willingness to increase their running volume. Finally, you can boost your aerobic fitness by doing longer long runs next year. I consider this option a good one for any runner who was limited by his or her aerobic fitness and is not already doing the longest long runs that are sensible with respect to his or her peak-race distance.

Was I limited by my neuromuscular fitness?

There are three major signs that you lacked adequate neuromuscular fitness in the past year. The first two are more or less the opposite of the first two signs of inadequate aerobic fitness mentioned above. If you tended to perform best in your longest races and worst in your shortest ones, and/or if you tended to feel stronger in longer, slower workouts than you did in shorter, faster workouts, your neuromuscular fitness was probably a limiter. A third indicator of limiting neuromuscular fitness is injuries or problems with muscle and tendon soreness.

The best way to address limiting neuromuscular fitness in planning next year's training depends on precisely how it limited you last year. If you feel that you simply lacked adequate speed and power, add more hill sprints and more interval work at 1,500-meter to 3K pace to your training. This doesn't necessarily mean you have to do a greater total amount of speed and power training in the early fundamental period, when this type of training receives its greatest emphasis. It might just mean that you train for speed and power more consistently throughout the training cycle by introducing it earlier and by not deemphasizing it as much in the later stages of the training cycle.

If you feel that you lacked strength more than you lacked raw sprint speed and power, the best response is to add some additional uphill running to your training next year. Specifically, run more hill repetitions, especially at the beginning of the fundamental period. In the remainder of the training cycle, transfer some of the interval work you would normally do on level ground to hills.

Hills are also my prescription to correct problems with injuries and soreness. If you had these problems last year, increase your commitment to steep hill sprints next year by doing more total sprints each week and by doing them more consistently throughout the training cycle. This will enhance the strength of your running muscles and connective tissues, making them more injury-resistant. You might also benefit from transferring some of the interval work you would normally perform on level ground to hills. This will allow you to build speed with less stress on the legs.

Was I limited by my specific endurance?

If your aerobic or neuromuscular fitness level is lower than it should be, your specific-endurance fitness will suffer as well, because specific endurance is nothing more than a goal-specific combination of aerobic and neuromuscular fitness. But it is possible to have well-developed aerobic and neuromuscular fitness and still be limited by your specific endurance. This problem results from a failure to combine your aerobic and neuromuscular fitness in the appropriate way for your peak-race distance and goal time.

Suppose you're training for a 10K peak race. Your training program includes a fairly high volume of easy running, weekly long runs, and healthy doses of hill sprints and short intervals at 1,500-meter to 3K pace. But it does not include threshold runs or 10K-pace intervals—the workouts that are most specific to 10K racing. In this case you will reach a level of fitness that enables you to perform very well in your hill sprints, short intervals, and long runs, and you will probably run a decent 10K, too. But you will not perform as well in your peak race as you would if you included more specific-endurance work in your training.

If you had a disappointing peak race last year despite performing well in your speed work and long runs during the latter weeks of training, then you were most likely limited by your specific endurance. The same diagnosis can be made if you tended to feel stronger in workouts in which you ran substantially faster or slower than race pace than you did in workouts run at or near race pace. And if you simply did not do much race-pace running last year, you can be sure you were limited by your specific endurance even in the absence of other signs.

The cure for a diagnosis of limiting specific endurance is obvious. Do more specific-endurance training next year! Be sure to introduce a small amount of specific-endurance work, in the form of fartlek intervals and/or progressions (depending on your peak-race distance), at the beginning of the training cycle. Gradually increase the amount of specific-endurance training throughout the training cycle. In the sharpening period, all three of your weekly hard workouts should be highly race-specific.

Experimentation

Everything you do in training is an experiment, and it should all be viewed as such. You never know exactly how your body will respond to any specific workout or training pattern. Your expectations for how your body will respond are nothing more than a hypothesis. When your body's actual response to training differs from your expectations, you must revise your hypothesis and tweak your future training accordingly. Too often, runners hang on to their hypotheses concerning the workouts and training patterns that ought to work best for them even after their application disproves them. Don't make this mistake! When a given training practice does not work as well as expected, try a new one.

There is, of course, a converse aspect to this principle. When a given training practice does work for you, it's important that you retain it. But competitive runners are much more likely to retain familiar practices that don't work than to discard proven practices that do.

The fact that a certain training practice appears to give you good results does not mean that an alternative practice might not give you even better results, however. For this reason, I recommend that you stay open to experimentation even when you feel that everything in your training is working. There is no such thing as perfect training. The concept of perfection implies permanence and stasis. But in the process of training for distance running, your body is constantly changing. Consequently, training patterns that seem perfect for you now will no longer be perfect for you next year, or even next month. If you train exactly the same way next year or next month, you will not improve as much as you would if you took account of changes in your running fitness and modified your training appropriately.

I am not talking about drastic changes. Once you have begun to practice adaptive running, there will be no more need for drastic changes in your training. But there are plenty of minor changes you can make that will have a measurable impact on your progress as a runner. These minor changes are mainly to be found at the level of workout formats. There is a whole universe of specific workout formats out there. This book contains only a fraction of them. I encourage you to continuously learn about other workouts and try those that are compatible with the adaptive running system and seem to offer some potential to improve your performance.

I try new workouts on my runners all the time. Recently I borrowed a new workout from Nic Bideau, who coaches the Australian runner Craig Mottram. The workout starts (following a warm-up, of course) with six laps around the track. The first lap is typically run at 10K pace or slightly slower. Each subsequent lap is a little faster. The sixth lap is run at 3K to 1,500-meter pace. The runner then jogs a lap and completes a set of eight 200-meter intervals at 5K to 3K pace with 100-meter active recoveries after each. This entire sequence is then repeated. (If you choose to try this workout, you will probably want to complete the sequence just one time.) I like this workout because it allows my runners to perform a fairly large amount of work in a way that is not too taxing. Also, it can be adjusted for use at any point in the training cycle through manipulation of the pace targets.

It's best to experiment in a controlled way. I don't recommend trying new workouts too frequently or testing multiple new workouts simultaneously. As important as adaptability is in training, structure is also important. The single most important characteristic of a training cycle is *direction*. It has to move consistently in the direction of race-specific fitness. It's very difficult to ensure that your training is doing this if you are constantly changing things. To ensure that they are truly building on each other, your workouts must maintain a "family resemblance" throughout the training process, changing only within certain strict parameters. Once you've settled on the types of workouts you plan to do in your next training cycle, it's best to stick with them, modifying only the details based on how your body responds. Thus, the best time to select new workouts to try is between training cycles, when you're planning and have not yet started the next ramp-up toward a peak race.

Setting Higher Goals

Suppose I challenged you to run as far as you could at a certain pace. My instructions were to hang on at the designated pace until you were so exhausted that you could not take another single stride without slowing down. Now let's suppose you were able to run 13.91 miles at this pace before throwing in the towel. Knowing this, I could almost guarantee that if I had challenged you not to run as far as you could at that pace, but to run 14 miles at the same pace, you could have done it, because that objective goal would have motivated you to push through a little more suffering than you believed you could overcome without the goal.

This little thought experiment is intended to make the point that it is impossible to produce a truly maximal race effort without chasing some type of goal, whether it's beating another runner to the finish line or beating a personal best time for the distance. You might think you're running as hard as you can when you race without any particular goal established, but you're not. It's an unalterable reality of how the mind affects the body during running.

Naturally, the mind can overcome only so much matter. You cannot achieve just any goal simply by setting it. Going back to the thought experiment described above, if I had challenged you to run 15 miles at the designated pace, knowing that you could only run 13.91 miles without a goal, chances are very slim that you could have run an extra 1.09 miles without slowing down. An appropriate goal challenges you to push just a little bit harder than you otherwise would—to squeeze the last 1 percent of reserve that your mind allows your body to hold back without such a demand.

Past race performances provide the best information to use in setting appropriate future race goals. In most cases, next year's goal time for a given race distance should be slightly faster than the best time you achieved for that distance last year. Accumulating fitness and better training will render your body able to perform at a higher level next year, but you might not fully realize the potential of these changes unless you set goals that demand it. In other words, on top of everything else discussed in this chapter, *improvement requires that you aim for improvement*. When setting goals for next year, try to account for not only accumulating fitness and better training, but also for the need to reach higher in your mind so that your body can follow.

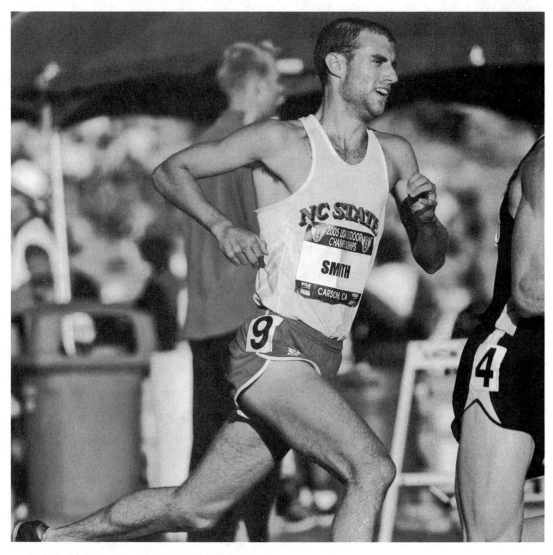

Andy Smith © Courtesy of the New York Road Runners

Runner Profile: Andy Smith

A lot of the runners I coach come to me as hard-luck cases—athletes whose careers have been stymied by frequent or major injury setbacks. Andy Smith might be the greatest hard-luck case of all. A 2005 graduate of North Carolina State University, Andy had only been able to run one race in two years due to injuries that culminated in surgery for compartment syndrome.

My work with Andy began with post-surgery rehabilitation in the early spring of 2007. My primary goal was to gradually and steadily increase his running volume to the point at which he was running twice a day and at least 100 miles per week. I was confident that by cautiously transforming Andy into a high-mileage runner I could greatly increase his durability and resilience.

In college, Andy had trained on the Lydiard system, which is characterized by lots of hard aerobic runs and very distinct training phases. I had him reduce the intensity of his aerobic running so that he could handle a much greater volume of such running, which was necessary to stimulate further aerobic development. Also, as I do with every runner, I made Andy's training more consistently well rounded, introducing hill sprints and small amounts of specific-endurance work as soon after his surgery as I felt it was safe to do so and steadily increasing the balance of his training from there.

Andy's primary event is the 3,000-meter steeplechase. Just eight weeks after his surgery, Andy ran an 8:34 steeplechase—just five seconds off his personal best time from college. Two weeks later he posted a personal best time of 13:38 for 5,000 meters. The future looks bright for this former hard-luck case.

The Self-Coaching Journey

10

We've covered a lot of ground in the preceding pages. The finish line is almost within sight. The next chapter is an "optional read" for youth and masters runners. The final chapter presents a selection of training plans that you may or may not choose to follow, or that you may choose to follow more or less exactly. You have already learned almost everything this book teaches about my adaptive running system. The time to start practicing it is drawing near. So, now what?

Let me begin to answer this question by telling you what would happen if you moved to Eugene, Oregon, and I began coaching you directly. The process would start with my asking you a lot of questions. These questions would fall into two general categories: (1) questions about your past as a runner, and (2) questions about the future you envision for yourself as a runner. Before I could take any sensible action as your coach, I would need to pick your brain for a good deal of information in these two general categories. The first steps we took together as a coach-athlete team would be designed to build on your past running and move in the direction of your short-term and long-term future goals.

These initial steps might be very different for you than they would be for another runner. I might increase your running volume while slightly reducing another runner's volume, or vice versa. I might have you do less speed work and more threshold work while having another runner do more specific-endurance work and less easy running. It all depends on the details of your respective running experience and goals.

Nevertheless, there would be some similarities. For both you and this hypothetical other runner, the primary objective of the first several weeks of training under my guidance would be simply to get accustomed to the adaptive running methods described in detail in chapter 2. These methods include the standard weekly workout schedule presented on page 146, steep-hill sprints, and very slow recovery runs. While the specific mix of workouts I gave you would be the blend that I expected to work best for you, we could not possibly predict exactly how your body would respond to them. Therefore these first weeks would also be a period of intense information gathering. We would closely monitor your performance in workouts, your fatigue level, and your aches and pains, and make any necessary adjustments based on these observations.

Except in the unlikely event that you developed an early injury or illness, these corrections would not be drastic, but they could be important. For example, we might find that you did not perform well in your Sunday long runs due to inadequate recovery from Friday's specific-endurance and speed workouts. In response to this observation, we might move your specific-endurance and speed workouts from Friday to Tuesday and move Tuesday's threshold runs, which you seem to recover from more quickly, from Tuesday to Friday.

This cycle of executing planned training, observing the results, and making small corrections based on the specific results we observed would continue until you ran your next peak race. After this race was completed we would measure your performance against our expectations, look back at the entire training cycle leading up to that race, and try to draw larger conclusions about what we did right, what we did wrong, and how we should change your training in the next training cycle.

The whole experience, as you can see, is one long experiment. If you came to me for coaching with the expectation that I would instantly know exactly what to do with you and "just do it," you would be very disappointed. Everything I know about running suffices only to help runners start on the right foot and continually learn from their training and racing, and improve based on this learning. And the greatest amount of learning comes from failures, setbacks, and disappointments, which you would be sure to experience with me as your coach.

This pattern applies to every runner I have ever coached, including the very best runners. Dathan Ritzenhein's first marathon is a good example. His 11th-place finish and 2:14:01 finishing time in the 2006 New York City Marathon were big disappointments when measured against our expectations. Together we looked closely at this race and the preceding training and tried to identify where we took a wrong turn. We decided that the problem was not any single major wrong turn but rather a number of smaller missteps. There was evidence that Dathan actually peaked two weeks early (he ran phenomenal workouts and felt unstoppable at this time, but then began slipping), so we took steps to delay his peak in preparation for the 2008 U.S. Olympic Team Trials–Men's Marathon, which was his next attempt at the 26.2-mile distance. We also felt that Dathan needed more raw endurance, so we included more long runs in the 20- to 24-mile range in his second marathon ramp-up. Also, based on the fact that Dathan did not consume any nutrition after the three-mile mark of his first marathon, we came to the obvious conclusion that he needed to take in more fluid and more energy in the Olympic Trials, so we had him practice consuming carbohydrate gels and water in his longer race-pace workouts and stick to a strict schedule of gel and water consumption in the race. It all paid off. Dathan ran a time of 2:11:07 on a much tougher course and claimed a slot on the Olympic team with a second-place finish.

When you finish reading this book and begin to practice adaptive running, you will move through a process that looks very much like the process I just described, in which we imagined that I began coaching you one-on-one. The information in this book will substitute for the knowledge in my head that I would apply in coaching you directly. Refer back to these pages as often as necessary as you proceed through your self-coaching journey. The more important functions of my role as a coach—monitoring my athletes' response to workouts, analyzing their workout and race results, and planning future training on the basis of this monitoring and analysis—are functions that you will have to fulfill on your own behalf. But it does not take any special skill to do these things. They are simply habits that you will practice with increasing effectiveness as you gain experience. Again, all of the guidelines you need to begin building these habits are contained in this book.

The most important consideration to keep in mind when taking your first steps in practicing adaptive running is that this training system is very much a step-by-step process. The first step, as I suggested above, is simply to try the core methods of the system and see how you respond. Don't burden yourself by thinking beyond this initial test. The time to look farther ahead is after you have gathered enough experience in practicing the adaptive running methods to have a good sense of what is working and what is not working, so you can base your planning on these observations rather than on some abstract ideas about what ought to work for you. This cycle of training, analyzing, and adjusting will continue indefinitely, just as it does for my runners and me. At first you may feel you're groping in the dark, exactly as I do when I begin working with a new athlete. The longer you coach yourself, the more confident and competent you will become in this role, but you will never achieve full mastery. You will continue to learn, and to adapt based on what you learn, and to improve thanks to your adaptability.

Running Faster

The goal of every competitive runner is to run faster. Achieving this goal, by setting a new personal best race time every now and again, is one of the most rewarding experiences in the life of the competitive runner. It would be a lot less satisfying, though, if running faster was totally predictable—if we always knew exactly what we needed to do to improve, so that actually improving was strictly a matter of going out and doing it. Improvement is quite predictable for beginning runners, naturally, but once your race times have progressed to a certain level and you have passed a certain threshold of training volume, figuring out how to stimulate further improvement becomes as challenging as the workouts themselves. I like it that way. The difficulty of discovering how to run faster lends the sport an exciting intellectual dimension and makes those hard-won moments of running faster all the more rewarding.

The art of coaching, and of self-coaching, is fundamentally a matter of taking a systematic approach to training that makes better performance more or less inevitable, if not entirely predictable. It begins with the premise that you cannot predict the future—or, specifically, how your body will respond to training. Therefore every workout is treated as an experiment. You then allow the results of these experiments to guide you toward a future of running faster. Training patterns that seem to hold you back are eliminated while those that seem to push you forward are kept and possibly increased or intensified. Sooner or later, this approach is bound to lead you to new personal best performances.

I like to draw an analogy between the way adaptive running yields personal records and the way world records are continually lowered over the years. No one can predict when a world record in a major running event such as the marathon will be broken, but we know that the existing record will be broken sooner or later. History leaves no doubt about it. The men's marathon world record has been broken 29 times since 1913, and the women's world record has been broken an equal number of times since 1964. Table 10.1 shows the specific progressions.

Table 10.1 Progression of Men's and Women's Marathon World Records

The men's marathon world record has been broken approximately once every 3.25 years over the past century. The women's marathon world record has been broken roughly once every 1.5 years since the event was first contested less than half a century ago.

Men		Women	
Time	Date	Time	Date
2:36:06	5-31-1913	3:27:45	5-23-1964
2:32:35	8-20-1920	3:19:33	7-21-1964
2:29:01	10-13-1925	3:15:22	5-6-1967
2:27:49	3-31-1935	3:07:26	9-16-1967
2:26:44	4-3-1935	3:02:53	2-28-1970
2:26:42	11-3-1935	3:01:42	5-9-1971
2:25:39	4-19-1947	2:55:22	9-19-1971
2:20:42	6-14-1952	2:49:40	12-5-1971
2:18:40	7-13-1953	2:46:36	12-2-1973
2:18:34	10-4-1953	2:46:24	10-27-1974
2:17:39	7-26-1954	2:43:54	12-1-1974
2:15:17	8-24-1958	2:42:24	4-21-1975
2:15:16	9-10-1960	2:40:15	5-3-1975
2:15:15	2-17-1963	2:38:19	10-12-1975
2:14:28	7-15-1963	2:35:15	5-1-1977
2:13:55	7-13-1964	2:34:47	9-10-1977
2:12:11	10-21-1964	2:32:29	10-22-1978
2:12:00	6-12-1965	2:27:32	10-21-1979
2:09:36	12-3-1967	2:25:41	10-26-1980
2:08:33	5-3-1969	2:25:29	10-25-1981
2:08:18	12-6-1981	2:25:28	4-17-1983
2:08:05	10-21-1984	2:22:43	4-18-1983
2:07:12	4-20-1985	2:21:06	4-21-1985
2:06:50	4-17-1988	2:20:47	4-19-1998
2:06:05	9-20-1998	2:20:43	9-26-1999
2:05:42	10-24-1999	2:19:46	9-30-2001
2:05:38	4-14-2002	2:18:47	10-7-2001
2:04:55	9-28-2003	2:17:18	10-13-2002
2:04:26	9-30-2007	2:15:25	4-13-2003

How is it that the breaking of world records is inevitable yet unpredictable? And for that matter, how is it that human beings keep managing to improve the historical best times in standard running events such as the marathon? The answer to both questions is that the worldwide sport of distance running is itself an adaptive system that is perfectly designed to push back the limits of human performance. When a runner sets a new world record, other elite runners begin to emulate the training practices and other factors associated with that performance, beginning with simply *aiming* for the new world best time in future races. The result is an evolutionary process by which innovative and superior practices spread throughout the population of competitive runners, becoming standard.

A very simple example has to do with the races in which marathon world records are broken. The world record performances listed in the top half of table 10.1 took place in a wide variety of different marathon events, many of which featured less than ideal courses for world record setting. The world record performances in the bottom half of the table came from just a handful of events: the London, Chicago, Rotterdam, and Berlin marathons, all of which feature pancake-flat courses and "rabbits" (or pacesetters) to facilitate fast times. The sport of distance running has passed beyond the evolutionary stage at which it was possible to set a world record on a course with significant hills, such as the New York City Marathon (where the women's world record was broken four straight years between 1978 and 1981).

If we looked behind the race performances at the training of world record breakers we would see a similar evolutionary process. The most basic adaptation is increasing training mileage. Grete Waitz ran only 70 miles per week prior to breaking the marathon world record in 1978. The current world record holder, Paula Radcliffe, ran 150 miles per week in preparing for her all-time best performance. The marathon world record will never again be broken by someone who trains much less than this amount.

The factor that makes world records unpredictable, despite their inevitability, is the accidental nature of the innovations that make better performances possible. Innovations such as altitude training, cross-training, sports drinks, and elite running teams have undoubtedly contributed to the downward march of marathon world record times, yet their effects and even their emergence were entirely unforeseeable. Each of these innovations, as well as most innovations in specific training practices, came about as the result of a single person or a small group of people simply trying something that worked, and then spread throughout the sport.

Your quest to run faster than you've ever run before will closely parallel the process by which humanity continually redefines the limits of human running performance. Your journey as a self-coached runner using the adaptive running system will involve the same process of experimentation leading to adaptation and better performance. The parameters are much narrower for you, of course, as they are for any runner in comparison to the full history of the sport of distance running. Your innovations are more likely to consist in making small refinements to your training based on your progress and accumulated experience rather than in discovering things like altitude training and sports drinks. But the basic game is the same. Try stuff. See how it goes. Do more of what improves your running and less of what does not. This is the recipe for running faster at all levels of the sport—all the way from the first person across the finish line to the last. You might not be accustomed to comparing yourself to world record breakers, but you'll get used to it.

Adaptive Running for Youth and Masters Runners

11

A 15-year-old runner should not train the same way that a 25-year old runner does. Likewise, a 65-year-old runner should not—and in all probability cannot—train the same way that either a 15-year-old runner or a 25-year-old runner does. Our bodies change dramatically over the course of our lives. Since the adaptive running system is based on the principle that one's training must be customized to one's own body, it follows that youth runners (under 20) and masters runners (over 40) need to practice adaptive running somewhat differently than those in the middle.

Youth runners are, by virtue of their age, relatively new to running, and not only to running but also to exercise in general. For this reason, the primary focus of their training should be to develop a foundation of aerobic fitness and neuromuscular fitness from the most basic level. The first step in the long process of developing a lifetime-peak level of aerobic fitness is to gradually inure the body to increasing mileage. There is little to be gained at this point from more advanced types of aerobic training such as longer threshold runs or faster long runs. Almost all of the running that youth runners do should occur at an easy pace, which facilitates increasing mileage better than hard running does.

The first step in developing neuromuscular fitness is to perform a small number of very short, maximal-intensity efforts. As you know, I believe that the safest and most effective form of maximal-intensity training for all runners is short hill sprints. Youth runners should also work on developing balanced muscle strength throughout their bodies by engaging in regular resistance training—particularly core-muscle work—and participating in other sports, such as basketball and soccer. These efforts to develop whole-body muscle balance will pay off in the future by reducing injury risk when the runner focuses on running and trains at a high level as an adult.

The major difference between the bodies of youth runners and those of masters runners is that the bodies of youth runners are much more resilient. They adapt to and recover from training stress faster. Consequently, youth runners can increase their training workload faster and, eventually, handle a greater overall training workload. Properly trained older runners can handle hard workouts, but they cannot do them as often as younger runners can.

The muscles and connective tissues of masters runners are less elastic than those of youth runners. Tissue elasticity plays a critical role in enhancing running economy, because it enables runners to capture energy provided by impact forces and reuse it by directing it back into the ground. There is some evidence that years of high-volume running accelerate the age-related decline in elasticity of the muscles and connective tissues of the legs. This may explain why most of the distance-running world records in the older age categories (age 50 and beyond) are held by individuals who began running rather late in life. In any case, older runners need to train efficiently—focusing on "big-bang-for-the-buck" workouts and minimizing "filler" workouts—in order to minimize the negative effects of repetitive impact on tissue elasticity in their legs.

Joint mobility and muscle strength also tend to decline with age. You can slow this process drastically through mobility training and strength training. These types of cross-training are beneficial to runners of every age, but they are especially helpful to older runners.

In view of all of these aging factors—slower recovery and adaptation, declining tissue elasticity, and declining mobility and strength—I recommend that masters runners take a cross-training-based approach to training. In this approach, one runs only three or four times per week; most or all of these runs are harder workouts; and the running schedule is supplemented with nonimpact cardio cross-training, mobility training, and strength training.

In this chapter, I will present four training plans for youth runners and a pair of training plans for masters runners. Because most youth runners follow training programs overseen by their coaches during the school year, my youth training plans are summer base-training plans designed to get high school runners in shape for the cross-country season. The two masters training plans are road-race–focused. The first culminates in a 10K peak race, the second in a marathon peak race. In addition to being useful in themselves, these plans can serve as general models that you can use to modify any of the training plans presented in the next chapter to make them better suited to masters runners.

Workout Key

The training plans themselves provide most of the information that you'll need to do each workout correctly. The following workout key provides supplementary guidelines for some of the workouts prescribed in the four youth training plans and the two masters training plans.

Easy Run—Run the prescribed distance at a natural, comfortable pace.

Hill Sprints—Run the prescribed distance at maximal effort up a steep hill. Recover by walking back down. Complete the prescribed number of repetitions. Start your hill sprints as soon as you finish your easy run.

X-Train—Cross-train in a nonimpact aerobic activity such as bicycling or elliptical training. Mimic the intensity of your easy runs.

Core Workout/Strength—Perform five or six exercises to strengthen the muscles of the hips, buttocks, abdomen, lower back, and upper torso.

Fartlek Run—Run the first and last miles of the prescribed workout at your easy-run pace. Also run the middle segment at your easy-run pace, but accelerate to the designated interval pace for the prescribed duration and number of fartlek intervals. These intervals do not need to be evenly spaced out, but allow enough active recovery time after each to ensure that you're ready for the next.

Strides—Do these short intervals at 1,500-meter pace immediately after finishing your easy run. Recover by jogging back to your starting point.

Drills—See pages 88–90.

Progression Run—Start the run at your easy-run pace. Do the last portion at either a "moderate" effort (an effort that feels moderately hard relative to the distance) or a "hard" effort (an effort that feels hard but manageable relative to the distance). Do uphill progressions on a long, steady, moderate incline (or on a treadmill set at a 4- to 6-percent incline), if possible. Do all other progressions on flat or relatively flat terrain.

Long Run—Sunday runs are designated as long runs by default in these schedules, regardless of their length, because "long" is relative and Sunday is set aside as a day for endurance-building stimuli in the adaptive running system. Even when they are only four or five miles, long runs are almost always as long as, or longer than, any other run in the same week.

Training Plans for Youth Runners

In this section I present four summer base-training plans for youth runners. Each is 12 weeks long. The "Freshman Plan" peaks at 26 miles per week, the "Sophomore Plan" at 39 miles per week, the "Junior Plan" at 54 miles per week, and the "Senior Plan"—for serious and experienced high school runners—at 70 miles per week.

The Freshman Plan							
Week #	Sunday	Monday	Tuesday	Wednesday	Thursday	Friday	Saturday
1	Rest	Easy Run 3 miles Core Workout	Easy Run 3 miles + 1 × 8-sec. hill sprint	X-Train 20 minutes or Rest	Easy Run 3 miles Core Workout	Easy Run 3 miles + 1 × 8-sec. hill sprint	X-Train 20 minutes or Rest
2	Rest	Easy Run 4 miles Core Workout	Easy Run 3 miles + 2 × 8-sec. hill sprint	X-Train 20 minutes or Rest	Easy Run 3 miles Core Workout	Easy Run 4 miles + 2 × 8-sec. hill sprint	X-Train 20 minutes or Rest
3	Rest	Easy Run 5 miles Core Workout	Easy Run 3 miles + 3 × 8-sec. hill sprint	X-Train 25 minutes or Rest	Easy Run 3 miles Core Workout	Easy Run 5 miles + 3 × 8-sec. hill sprint	X-Train 25 minutes or Rest
4	Rest	Easy Run 5 miles Core Workout	Easy Run 4 miles + 5 × 8-sec. hill sprint	X-Train 25 minutes or Rest	Easy Run 3 miles Core Workout	Easy Run 5 miles + 5 × 8-sec. hill sprint	X-Train 25 minutes or Rest
5	Rest	Easy Run 6 miles Core Workout	Easy Run 4 miles + 5 × 8-sec. hill sprint	X-Train 30 minutes or Rest	Easy Run 4 miles Core Workout	Easy Run 6 miles + 5 × 8-sec. hill sprint	X-Train 30 minutes or Rest
6	Rest	Easy Run 6 miles Core Workout	Easy Run 5 miles + 6 × 8-sec. hill sprint	X-Train 30 minutes or Rest	Easy Run 4 miles Core Workout	Easy Run 6 miles + 6 × 8-sec. hill sprint	X-Train 30 minutes or Rest
7	Rest	Easy Run 7 miles Core Workout	Easy Run 5 miles + 7 × 8-sec. hill sprint	X-Train 35 minutes or Rest	Fartlek Run 6 miles easy w/4–6 × 30 sec. @ 5K pace Core Workout	Easy Run 5 miles + 7 × 8-sec. hill sprint	X-Train 35 minutes or Rest

Week #	Sunday	Monday	Tuesday	Wednesday	Thursday	Friday	Saturday
8	Rest	Easy Run 7 miles Core Workout	Easy Run 5 miles + 8 × 8-sec. hill sprint	X-Train 35 minutes or Rest	Fartlek Run 6 miles easy w/6–8 × 30 sec. @ 5K pace Core Workout	Easy Run 6 miles + drills (1 set)	X-Train 35 minutes or Rest
9	Rest	Easy Run 7 miles Core Workout	Easy Run 5 miles + 10 × 8-sec. hill sprint	X-Train 40 minutes or Rest	Fartlek Run 6 miles easy w/6–8 × 35 sec. @ 5K pace Core Workout	Easy Run 6 miles + drills (2 sets)	X-Train 40 minutes or Rest
10	Rest	Easy Run 7 miles Core Workout	Easy Run 5 miles + 10 × 8-sec. hill sprint	X-Train 40 minutes or Rest	Fartlek Run 5 miles easy w/4–6 × 40 sec. @ 5K pace Core Workout	Easy Run 6 miles + drills (3 sets)	Time Trial 1 mile easy 3 × 100m strides 5K time trial 1 mile easy
11	Rest	Easy Run 7 miles Core Workout	Easy Run 5 miles + 10 × 8-sec. hill sprint	X-Train 40 minutes or Rest	Fartlek Run 6 miles easy w/6–8 × 40 sec. @ 5K pace Core Workout	Easy Run 4 miles + drills (3 sets)	Easy Run 3 miles
12	Rest	Easy Run 7 miles Core Workout	Easy Run 5 miles + 10 × 8-sec. hill sprint	X-Train 40 minutes or Rest	Fartlek Run 6 miles easy w/6–8 × 45 sec. @ 5K pace Core Workout	Easy Run 4 miles + drills (3 sets)	Easy Run 4 miles

The Sophomore Plan

Week #	Sunday	Monday	Tuesday	Wednesday	Thursday	Friday	Saturday
1	Long Run 4 miles easy Core Workout	Rest	Easy Run 4 miles + 1 × 8-sec. hill sprint	X-Train 20 minutes or Rest	Easy Run 4 miles Core Workout	X-Train 20 minutes or Rest	Easy Run 3 miles + 1 × 8-sec. hill sprint
2	Long Run 5 miles easy Core Workout	Rest	Easy Run 4 miles + 2 × 8-sec. hill sprint	X-Train 20 minutes or Rest	Easy Run 4 miles Core Workout	X-Train 20 minutes or Rest	Easy Run 4 miles + 2 × 8-sec. hill sprint
3	Long Run 6 miles easy Core Workout	Rest	Easy Run 5 miles + 3 × 8-sec. hill sprint	X-Train 25 minutes or Rest	Easy Run 6 miles Core Workout	X-Train 25 minutes or Rest	Easy Run 5 miles + 3 × 8-sec. hill sprint
4	Long Run 6 miles easy Core Workout	Rest	Easy Run 6 miles + 4 × 8-sec. hill sprint	X-Train 25 minutes or Rest	Easy Run 6 miles Core Workout	Easy Run 3 miles	Easy Run 4 miles + 4 × 8-sec. hill sprint
5	Long Run 7 miles easy Core Workout	Rest	Easy Run 6 miles + 5 × 8-sec. hill sprint	Easy Run 5 miles	Easy Run 5 miles Core Workout	X-Train 30 minutes or Rest	Easy Run 5 miles + 5 × 8-sec. hill sprint
6	Long Run 7 miles easy Core Workout	Easy Run 6 miles + 6 × 8-sec. hill sprint	X-Train 30 minutes or Rest	Easy Run 7 miles	Fartlek Run 6 miles easy w/6–8 × 30 sec. @ 5K pace Core Workout	X-Train 30 minutes or Rest	Easy Run 5 miles + 6 × 8-sec. hill sprint
7	Long Run 8 miles easy Core Workout	Easy Run 6 miles + 7 × 8-sec. hill sprint	X-Train 35 minutes or Rest	Easy Run 7 miles + drills (1 set)	Fartlek Run 6 miles easy w/8–10 × 30 sec. @ 5K pace Core Workout	X-Train 35 minutes or Rest	Easy Run 4 miles + 7 × 8-sec. hill sprint

Week #	Sunday	Monday	Tuesday	Wednesday	Thursday	Friday	Saturday
8	Long Run 8 miles easy Core Workout	Easy Run 6 miles + 8 × 8-sec. hill sprint	X-Train 35 minutes or Rest	Easy Run 7 miles + drills (2 sets)	Fartlek Run 6 miles easy w/6–8 × 40 sec. @ 5K pace Core Workout	Easy Run 4 miles	Easy Run 4 miles + drills (2 sets)
9	Long Run 8 miles easy Core Workout	Easy Run 6 miles + 10 × 8-sec. hill sprint	X-Train 40 minutes or Rest	Easy Run 7 miles + drills (2 sets)	Fartlek Run 6 miles easy w/6–8 × 50 sec. @ 5K pace Core Workout	Easy Run 5 miles	Easy Run 4 miles + drills (2 sets)
10	Long Run 8 miles easy Core Workout	Easy Run 6 miles + 10 × 8-sec. hill sprint	X-Train 40 minutes or Rest	Easy Run 7 miles + drills (1 set)	Fartlek Run 6 miles easy w/6–8 × 50 sec. @ 5K pace Core Workout	Easy Run 6 miles	Easy Run 5 miles + drills (2 sets)
11	Long Run 8 miles easy Core Workout	Easy Run 6 miles + 10 × 8-sec. hill sprint	X-Train 45 minutes or Rest	Easy Run 7 miles + drills (1 set)	Fartlek Run 6 miles easy w/8–10 × 50 sec. @ 5K pace Core Workout	Easy Run 6 miles	Easy Run 5 miles + drills (2 sets)
12	Long Run 9 miles easy Core Workout	Easy Run 6 miles + 10 × 8-sec. hill sprint	X-Train 45 minutes or Rest	Easy Run 7 miles + drills (1 set)	Fartlek Run 6 miles easy w/8–10 × 50 sec. @ 5K pace Core Workout	Easy Run 6 miles	Easy Run 5 miles + drills (2 sets)

Chapter 11   Adaptive Running for Youth and Masters Runners   217

The Junior Plan							
Week #	Sunday	Monday	Tuesday	Wednesday	Thursday	Friday	Saturday
1	Long Run 5 miles easy Core Workout	Easy Run 4 miles + 1 × 8-sec. hill sprint	Easy Run 4 miles	Easy Run 4 miles Core Workout	Off	Easy Run 5 miles + 1 × 8-sec. hill sprint	Easy Run 3 miles
2	Long Run 6 miles easy Core Workout	Easy Run 5 miles + 2 × 8-sec. hill sprint	Easy Run 5 miles	Easy Run 5 miles Core Workout	Off	Easy Run 5 miles + 2 × 8-sec. hill sprint	Easy Run 3 miles
3	Long Run 6 miles easy Core Workout	Easy Run 5 miles + 3 × 8-sec. hill sprint	Easy Run 5 miles	Easy Run 5 miles Core Workout	Off	Easy Run 6 miles + 3 × 8-sec. hill sprint	Easy Run 3 miles
4	Long Run 7 miles easy Core Workout	Easy Run 5 miles + 4 × 8-sec. hill sprint	Easy Run 6 miles	Easy Run 7 miles Core Workout	Off	Easy Run 7 miles + 4 × 8-sec. hill sprint	Easy Run 4 miles
5	Long Run 7 miles easy Core Workout	Easy Run 6 miles + 5 × 8-sec. hill sprint	Easy Run 7 miles	Easy Run 7 miles Core Workout	Off	Easy Run 7 miles + 5 × 8-sec. hill sprint	Easy Run 4 miles
6	Progression Run 8 miles, last 15 min. moderate (uphill, if possible) Core Workout	Easy Run 6 miles + 6 × 8-sec. hill sprint	Easy Run 7 miles	Easy Run 8 miles w/4-mile moderate progression Core Workout	Off	Easy Run 8 miles + 6 × 8-sec. hill sprint	Easy Run 4 miles
7	Progression Run 8 miles, last 20 min. moderate (uphill, if possible) Core Workout	Easy Run 6 miles + 7 × 8-sec. hill sprint	Easy Run 7 miles + drills (1 set)	Easy Run 7 miles w/3.5-mile moderate progression Core Workout	Off	Fartlek Run 6 miles easy w/6–8 × 30 sec. @ 5K race pace	Easy Run 4 miles + drills (1 set)

Week #	Sunday	Monday	Tuesday	Wednesday	Thursday	Friday	Saturday
8	Progression Run 9 miles, last 20 min. moderate (uphill, if possible) Core Workout	Easy Run 6 miles + 8 × 8-sec. hill sprint	Easy Run 7 miles + drills (2 sets)	Easy Run 8 miles w/4-mile moderate progression Core Workout	Off	Fartlek Run 7 miles easy w/6–8 × 35 sec. @ 5K race pace	Easy Run 4 miles + drills (2 sets)
9	Progression Run 9 miles, last 15 min. hard (uphill, if possible) Core Workout	Easy Run 6 miles + 10 × 8-sec. hill sprint	Easy Run 7 miles w/10-min. moderate progression + drills (2 sets)	Easy Run 7 miles w/3.5-mile moderate progression Core Workout	Off	Fartlek Run 8 miles easy w/6–8 × 40 sec. @ 5K race pace	Easy Run 5 miles + drills (2 sets)
10	Long Run 8 miles easy Core Workout	Easy Run 6 miles + 10 × 8-sec. hill sprint	Easy Run 7 miles w/15-min. moderate progression + drills (2 sets)	Easy Run 9 miles w/4.5-mile moderate progression Core Workout	Off	Fartlek Run 7 miles easy w/6–8 × 45 sec. @ 5K race pace	Easy Run 5 miles + drills (2 sets)
11	Progression Run 10 miles, last 15 min. moderate Core Workout	Easy Run 7 miles + 10 × 8-sec. hill sprint	Easy Run 8 miles + drills (3 sets)	Easy Run 9 miles Core Workout	Easy Run 4 miles	Fartlek Run 8 miles easy w/6–8 × 50 sec. @ 5K race pace	Easy Run 6 miles + drills (3 sets)
12	Progression Run 10 miles, last 15 min. hard Core Workout	Easy Run 7 miles + 10 × 8-sec. hill sprint	Easy Run 8 miles w/10-min. hard progression + drills (2 sets)	Easy/ Moderate Run 9 miles (4.5 miles easy, 4.5 miles moderate) Core Workout	Easy Run 6 miles	Fartlek Run 8 miles easy w/8–10 × 50 sec. @ 5K race pace	Easy Run 6 miles + drills (2 sets)

The Senior Plan							
Week #	Sunday	Monday	Tuesday	Wednesday	Thursday	Friday	Saturday
1	Long Run 6 miles easy	Easy Run 5 miles + 2 × 8-sec. hill sprint	Easy Run 5 miles Core Workout	Easy Run 6 miles	Easy Run 5 miles + 2 × 8-sec. hill sprint Core Workout	Easy Run 6 miles	Core Workout
2	Long Run 7 miles easy	Easy Run 5 miles + 4 × 8-sec. hill sprint	Easy Run 6 miles Core Workout	Easy Run 6 miles	Easy Run 5 miles + 4 × 8-sec. hill sprint Core Workout	Easy Run 6 miles	Core Workout
3	Long Run 6 miles easy	Easy Run 5 miles + 6 × 8-sec. hill sprint	Easy Run 5 miles Core Workout	Easy Run 7 miles	Easy Run 6 miles + 6 × 8-sec. hill sprint Core Workout	Easy Run 6 miles	Core Workout
4	Progression Run 7 miles, last 5 min. moderate (uphill, if possible)	Easy Run 5 miles + 8 × 8-sec. hill sprint	Easy Run 7 miles Core Workout	Easy Run 7 miles	Easy Run 6 miles + 8 × 8-sec. hill sprint Core Workout	Easy Run 7 miles	Very Easy Run 4 miles Core Workout
5	Progression Run 8 miles, last 5 min. moderate (uphill, if possible)	Easy Run 5 miles + 10 × 10-sec. hill sprint	Progression Run 7 miles Start easy, finish w/10-min. moderate progression Core Workout	Progression Run 8 miles (4 miles easy, 4 miles moderate)	Easy Run 7 miles + drills (1 set) Core Workout	Progression Run 8 miles Start easy, finish w/30-min. moderate progression	Very Easy Run 4 miles Core Workout

Week #	Sunday	Monday	Tuesday	Wednesday	Thursday	Friday	Saturday
6	Progression Run 9 miles, last 10 min. moderate (uphill, if possible)	Easy Run 6 miles + 10 × 10-sec. hill sprint	Progression Run 7 miles Start easy, finish w/15-min. moderate progression Core Workout	Progression Run 8 miles (4 miles easy, 4 miles moderate)	Easy Run 7 miles + drills (1 set) Core Workout	Fartlek Run 8 miles easy w/6–8 × 30 sec. @ 5K pace	Very Easy Run 4 miles Core Workout
7	Progression Run 10 miles, last 15 min. moderate (uphill, if possible)	Easy Run 7 miles + 10 × 10-sec. hill sprint	Progression Run 7 miles Start easy, finish w/15-min. moderate progression Core Workout	Progression Run 9 miles (4.5 miles easy, 4.5 miles moderate)	Easy Run 7 miles + drills (1 set) Core Workout	Fartlek Run 9 miles easy w/8–10 × 35 sec. @ 5K pace	Very Easy Run 4 miles Core Workout
8	Progression Run 11 miles, last 20 min. moderate (uphill, if possible)	Easy Run 7 miles + 10 × 12-sec. hill sprint	Progression Run 8 miles Start easy, finish w/15-min. moderate progression Core Workout	Progression Run 9 miles (4.5 miles easy, 4.5 miles moderate)	Easy Run 7 miles + drills (2 sets) Core Workout	Fartlek Run 9 miles easy w/8–10 × 40 sec. @ 5K pace	Very Easy Run 4 miles Core Workout
9	Progression Run 9 miles, last 10 min. hard (uphill, if possible)	Easy Run 7 miles + 10 × 12-sec. hill sprint	Progression Run 8 miles Start easy, finish w/20-min. hard progression Core Workout	Progression Run 10 miles (5 miles easy, 5 miles moderate)	Easy Run 7 miles + drills (2 sets) Core Workout	Fartlek Run 10 miles easy w/10–12 × 45 sec. @ 5K pace	Very Easy Run 4 miles Core Workout

Week #	Sunday	Monday	Tuesday	Wednesday	Thursday	Friday	Saturday
10	Progression Run 12 miles, last 10 min. hard (uphill, if possible)	Easy Run 8 miles + 10 × 12-sec. hill sprint	Progression Run 9 miles Start easy, finish w/20-min. hard progression Core Workout	Progression Run 10 miles (5 miles easy, 5 miles moderate)	Easy Run 7 miles + drills (2 sets) Core Workout	Fartlek Run 10 miles easy w/10–12 × 45 sec. @ 5K pace	Very Easy Run 4 miles Core Workout
11	Progression Run 13 miles, last 20 min. hard	Easy Run 5 miles + 10 × 12-sec. hill sprint Easy Run 4 miles	Progression Run 8 miles Start easy, finish w/20-min. hard progression Core Workout	Progression Run 11 miles (5.5 miles easy, 5.5 miles moderate)	Easy Run 7 miles + drills (2 sets) Core Workout	Fartlek Run 10 miles easy w/10–12 × 50 sec. @ 5K pace	Very Easy Run 4 miles Core Workout
12	Progression Run 14 miles, last 20 min. hard	Easy Run 5 miles + 10 × 12-sec. hill sprint Easy Run 5 miles	Progression Run 8 miles Start easy, finish w/25-min. hard progression Core Workout	Easy Run 5 miles Easy Run 5 miles	Easy Run 5 miles Easy Run 5 miles + drills (2 sets) Core Workout	Easy Run 4 miles Fartlek Run 10 miles easy w/10–12 × 50 sec. @ 5K pace	Very Easy Run 4 miles Core Workout

Training Plans for Masters Runners

In this section, I present a pair of training plans designed especially for masters runners. The first plan is a 16-week schedule culminating in a 10K peak race. The second is a 20-week schedule culminating in a marathon peak race. Both plans are cross-training–based and include only three running workouts per week.

Week #	Sunday	Monday	Tuesday	Wednesday	Thursday	Friday	Saturday
Masters 10K Training Plan							
1	Long Run 5 miles easy	Core Strength 1 set	Easy Run 4 miles + 1 × 8-sec. hill sprint	Core Strength 1 set	Fartlek Run 5 miles easy w/6 × 30 sec. intervals @ 10K–3K pace	Core Strength 1 set	X-Train 20 min.
2	Progression Run 6 miles easy, last mile moderate (uphill, if possible)	Core Strength 1 set	Easy Run 5 miles + 2 × 8-sec. hill sprint	Core Strength 1 set	Fartlek Run 6 miles easy w/6 × 40 sec. intervals @ 10K–3K pace	Core Strength 1 set	X-Train 25 min.
3	Progression Run 7 miles easy, last 1.5 miles moderate (uphill, if possible)	Core Strength 1 set	Easy Run 5 miles + 3 × 8-sec. hill sprint	Core Strength 1 set	Fartlek Run 7 miles easy w/8 × 40 sec. intervals @ 10K–3K pace	Core Strength 1 set	X-Train 30 min.
4	Progression Run 5.5 miles easy, last 1.5 miles moderate (uphill, if possible)	Core Strength 1 set	Easy Run 4 miles + 4 × 8-sec. hill sprint	Core Strength 1 set	Fartlek Run 5 miles easy w/6 × 30 sec. intervals @ 10K–3K pace	Core Strength 1 set	X-Train 20 min.
5	Progression Run 7 miles, last 2 miles moderate	Core Strength 2 sets	Anaerobic Hill Intervals 1 mile easy 4 × 400m uphill @ 3K effort w/2-min. active recoveries 1 mile easy + 5 × 8-sec. hill sprint	Core Strength 2 sets	Progression Run 4 miles easy + 2 miles hard (uphill, if possible)	Core Strength 2 sets	X-Train 30 min.

Week #	Sunday	Monday	Tuesday	Wednesday	Thursday	Friday	Saturday
6	Progression Run 7.5 miles, last 2.5 miles moderate	Core Strength 2 sets	Specific-Endurance Intervals 1 mile easy 5 × 1 mile @ current 10K pace w/2-min. active recoveries 1 mile easy + 6 × 8-sec. hill sprint	Core Strength 2 sets	Ladder Workout 1 mile easy 2 × (6 min., 5 min., 4 min., 3 min., 2 min., 1 min. @ 10K–1,500m pace w/2-min. active recoveries) 1 mile easy	Core Strength 2 sets	X-Train 35 min.
7	Progression Run 7 miles, last mile hard	Core Strength 2 sets	Anaerobic Hill Intervals 1 mile easy 4 × 600m uphill @ 3K effort w/2-min. active recoveries 1 mile easy + 7 × 8-sec. hill sprint	Core Strength 2 sets	Threshold Run 1 mile easy 2 miles @ half-marathon pace 1 mile easy 2 miles @ half-marathon pace 1 mile easy	Core Strength 2 sets	X-Train 40 min.
8	Progression Run 5 miles, last 2 miles moderate	Core Strength 2 sets	Speed Intervals 1 mile easy 6 × 400m @ 3K pace w/2-min. active recoveries 1 mile easy + 8 × 8-sec. hill sprint	Core Strength 2 sets	Threshold Run 1 mile easy 2 miles @ half-marathon pace 1 mile easy 1 mile @ 10K pace 1 mile easy	Core Strength 2 sets	X-Train 30 min.
9	Progression Run 7 miles, last 2 miles hard	Core Strength 2 sets	Ladder Workout 1 mile easy 2 × (6 min., 5 min., 4 min., 3 min., 2 min. 1 min. @ 10K–1,500m pace w/2-min. active recoveries) 1 mile easy + 9 × 8-sec. hill sprint	Core Strength 2 sets	Threshold Run 1 mile easy 2.5 miles @ half-marathon pace 1 mile easy 2.5 miles @ half-marathon pace 1 mile easy	Core Strength 2 sets	X-Train 40 min.

Week #	Sunday	Monday	Tuesday	Wednesday	Thursday	Friday	Saturday
10	Progression Run 8 miles, last 3 miles progressing moderate to hard	Core Strength 3 sets	Specific-Endurance Intervals 1 mile easy 8 × 1K @ goal 10K pace w/2-min. active recoveries 1 mile easy + 10 × 8-sec. hill sprint	Core Strength 3 sets	Threshold Run 1 mile easy 4 miles @ half-marathon pace 1 mile easy	Core Strength 3 sets	X-Train 45 min.
11	Progression Run 8.5 miles, last 3.5 miles progressing moderate to hard	Core Strength 3 sets	Specific-Endurance Intervals 1 mile easy 10 × 1K @ goal 10K pace w/2-min. active recoveries 1 mile easy + 8 × 10-sec. hill sprint	Core Strength 3 sets	Threshold Run 1 mile easy 3 miles @ half-marathon pace 1 mile easy 2 miles @ 10K pace 1 mile easy	Core Strength 3 sets	X-Train 50 min.
12	Progression Run 6 miles, last 2 miles progressing moderate to hard	Core Strength 3 sets	Specific-Endurance Intervals 1 mile easy 4 × 1 mile @ goal 10K pace w/2-min. active recoveries 1 mile easy + 8 × 10-sec. hill sprint	Core Strength 3 sets	Threshold Run 1 mile easy 2 miles @ half-marathon pace 1 mile easy 1 mile @ 10K pace 1 mile easy	Core Strength 3 sets	X-Train 40 min.
13	Hard Long Run 2 miles easy 2 miles @ half-marathon pace 1 mile easy 2 miles @ half-marathon pace 2 miles easy	Core Strength 3 sets	Specific-Endurance Intervals 1 mile easy 6 × 1 mile @ goal 10K pace w/2-min. active recoveries 1 mile easy + 8 × 10-sec. hill sprint	Core Strength 3 sets	Threshold Run 1 mile easy 3 miles @ half-marathon pace 1 mile easy 2 miles @ 10K pace 1 mile easy	Core Strength 3 sets	X-Train 50 min.

Week #	Sunday	Monday	Tuesday	Wednesday	Thursday	Friday	Saturday	
14	Hard Long Run 2 miles easy 2.5 miles @ half-marathon pace 1 mile easy 2.5 miles @ half-marathon pace 1 mile easy	Core Strength 2 sets	Specific-Endurance Intervals 1 mile easy 4 × 2K @ goal 10K pace w/2-min. active recoveries 1 mile easy + 10 × 10-sec. hill sprint	Core Strength 2 sets	Threshold Run 1 mile easy 3.5 miles @ half-marathon pace 1 mile easy 2.5 miles @ 10K pace 1 mile easy	Core Strength 2 sets	X-Train 55 min.	
15	Hard Long Run 1 mile easy 3 miles @ half-marathon pace 1 mile easy 3 miles @ half-marathon pace 1 mile easy	Core Strength 2 sets	Specific-Endurance Intervals 1 mile easy 4 × 2K @ goal 10K pace w/90-sec. active recoveries + 1K max effort 1 mile easy + 10 × 10-sec. hill sprint	Core Strength 2 sets	Threshold Run 1 mile easy 2 miles @ 10K pace 1 mile easy 2 miles @ 10K pace 1 mile easy	Core Strength 2 sets	X-Train 1 hour	
16	Hard Long Run 2 miles easy 4 miles @ half-marathon pace 2 miles easy	Core Strength 1 set	Specific-Endurance Intervals 1 mile easy 2 × 2K @ goal 10K pace w/2-min. active recoveries 1 mile easy + 4 × 10-sec. hill sprint	Core Strength 1 set	Threshold Run 1 mile easy 2 miles @ 10K pace 1 mile easy	Core Strength 1 set	Sa Off	Su 10K

Masters Marathon Plan							
Week #	Sunday	Monday	Tuesday	Wednesday	Thursday	Friday	Saturday
1	Long Run 6 miles easy	Core Strength 1 set	Easy Run 4 miles + 1 × 8-sec. hill sprint	Core Strength 1 set	Fartlek Run 5 miles easy w/6 × 30 sec. intervals @ 10K–3K pace	Core Strength 1 set	X-Train 20 min.
2	Long Run 7 miles easy	Core Strength 1 set	Easy Run 5 miles + 2 × 8-sec. hill sprint	Core Strength 1 set	Fartlek Run 6 miles easy w/6 × 40 sec. intervals @ 10K–3K pace	Core Strength 1 set	X-Train 25 min.
3	Long Run 8 miles easy	Core Strength 1 set	Easy Run 5 miles + 3 × 8-sec. hill sprint	Core Strength 1 set	Fartlek Run 7 miles easy w/8 × 40 sec. intervals @ 10K–3K pace	Core Strength 1 set	X-Train 30 min.
4	Long Run 6 miles easy	Core Strength 1 set	Easy Run 4 miles + 4 × 8-sec. hill sprint	Core Strength 1 set	Fartlek Run 5 miles easy w/6 × 30 sec. intervals @ 10K–3K pace	Core Strength 1 set	X-Train 20 min.
5	Progression Run 9 miles, last mile moderate (uphill, if possible)	Core Strength 2 sets	Anaerobic Hill Intervals 1 mile easy 4 × 400m uphill @ 3K effort w/2-min. active recoveries 1 mile easy + 5 × 8-sec. hill sprint	Core Strength 2 sets	Progression Run 4 miles easy + 2 miles hard (uphill, if possible)	Core Strength 2 sets	X-Train 30 min.
6	Progression Run 11 miles, last mile moderate (uphill, if possible)	Core Strength 2 sets	Anaerobic Hill Intervals 1 mile easy 4 × 600m uphill @ 3K effort w/2-min. active recoveries 1 mile easy + 6 × 8-sec. hill sprint	Core Strength 2 sets	Ladder Workout 1 mile easy 2 × (6 min., 5 min., 4 min., 3 min., 2 min., 1 min. @ 10K–1,500m pace w/2-min. active recoveries) 1 mile easy	Core Strength 2 sets	X-Train 35 min.

Week #	Sunday	Monday	Tuesday	Wednesday	Thursday	Friday	Saturday
7	Progression Run 13 miles, last 2 miles moderate (uphill, if possible)	Core Strength 2 sets	Ladder Workout 1 mile easy 1 mile, 1K, 800m, 400m, 200m w/400m jog recoveries @ 10K–1,500m pace + 7 × 8-sec. hill sprint	Core Strength 2 sets	Threshold Run 1 mile easy 2 miles @ half-marathon pace 1 mile easy 2 miles @ half-marathon pace 1 mile easy	Core Strength 2 sets	X-Train 40 min.
8	Long Run 8 miles easy	Core Strength 2 sets	Speed Intervals 1 mile easy 6 × 400m @ 3K pace w/2-min. active recoveries 1 mile easy + 8 × 8-sec. hill sprint	Core Strength 2 sets	Threshold Run 1 mile easy 2 miles @ half-marathon pace 1 mile easy 1 mile @ 10K pace 1 mile easy	Core Strength 2 sets	X-Train 30 min.
9	Progression Run 14 miles, last 2 miles moderate	Core Strength 2 sets	Anaerobic Hill Intervals 1 mile easy 5 × 600m uphill @ 3K effort w/2-min. active recoveries 1 mile easy + 9 × 8-sec. hill sprint	Core Strength 2 sets	Threshold Run 1 mile easy 2.5 miles @ half-marathon pace 1 mile easy 2.5 miles @ half-marathon pace 1 mile easy	Core Strength 2 sets	X-Train 40 min.
10	Progression Run 15 miles, last 3 miles moderate	Core Strength 3 sets	Speed Intervals 1 mile easy 8 × 400m @ 3K pace w/2-min. active recoveries 1 mile easy + 10 × 8-sec. hill sprint	Core Strength 3 sets	Threshold Run 1 mile easy 4 miles @ half-marathon pace 1 mile easy	Core Strength 3 sets	X-Train 45 min.

Week #	Sunday	Monday	Tuesday	Wednesday	Thursday	Friday	Saturday
11	Progression Run 16 miles, last 3 miles moderate	Core Strength 3 sets	Ladder Workout 1 mile easy 2 × (1 mile, 1K, 800m, 400m w/400m jog recoveries) @ 10K–1,500m pace + 8 × 10-sec. hill sprint	Core Strength 3 sets	Threshold Run 1 mile easy 3 miles @ half-marathon pace 1 mile easy 2 miles @ 10K pace 1 mile easy	Core Strength 3 sets	X-Train 50 min.
12	Progression Run 17 miles, last 3 miles progressing moderate to hard	Core Strength 3 sets	Specific-Endurance Intervals 1 mile easy 4 × 1 mile @ goal 10K pace w/2-min. active recoveries 1 mile easy + 8 × 10-sec. hill sprint	Core Strength 3 sets	Threshold Run 1 mile easy 2 miles @ half-marathon pace 1 mile easy 1 mile @ 10K pace 1 mile easy	Core Strength 1 set	10K Tune-Up Race
13	Long Run 8 miles easy	Core Strength 3 sets	Specific-Endurance Intervals 1 mile easy 5 × 1 mile @ goal 10K pace w/2-min. active recoveries 1 mile easy + 9 × 10-sec. hill sprint	Core Strength 3 sets	Threshold Run 1 mile easy 3 miles @ half-marathon pace 1 mile easy 2 miles @ 10K pace 1 mile easy	Core Strength 3 sets	X-Train 50 min.
14	Hard Long Run 14 miles easy 4 miles @ marathon pace	Core Strength 3 sets	Specific-Endurance Intervals 1 mile easy 5 × 1 mile @ goal 10K pace w/2-min. active recoveries 1 mile easy + 9 × 10-sec. hill sprint	Core Strength 3 sets	Threshold Run 1 mile easy 3.5 miles @ half-marathon pace 1 mile easy 2.5 miles @ 10K pace 1 mile easy	Core Strength 3 sets	X-Train 55 min.

Week #	Sunday	Monday	Tuesday	Wednesday	Thursday	Friday	Saturday
15	Marathon-Pace Run 6 miles easy + 5 × (1 mile @ marathon pace − 15 sec./mile, 1 mile @ marathon pace + 1 min./mile)	Core Strength 2 sets	Specific-Endurance Intervals 1 mile easy 5 × 1 mile @ goal 10K pace w/2-min. active recoveries 1 mile easy + 9 × 10-sec. hill sprint	Core Strength 2 sets	Threshold Run 1 mile easy 2 miles @ 10K pace 1 mile easy 2 miles @ 10K pace 1 mile easy	Core Strength 2 sets	X-Train 1 hour
16	Hard Long Run 16 miles easy 4 miles @ marathon pace	Core Strength 3 sets	Specific-Endurance Intervals 1 mile easy 2 × 2 miles @ half-marathon pace w/2-min. active recovery 1 mile easy + 4 × 10-sec. hill sprint	Core Strength 3 sets	Threshold Run 1 mile easy 2 miles @ 10K pace 1 mile easy	Core Strength 3 sets	Half-Marathon Tune-Up Race
17	Long Run 8 miles easy	Core Strength 3 sets	Specific-Endurance Intervals 1 mile easy 2 × 2 miles @ half-marathon pace w/2-min. active recovery 1 mile easy + 4 × 400m hills @ 3K effort	Core Strength 3 sets	Threshold Run 1 mile easy 2 miles @ marathon pace 0.5 mile easy 2 miles @ half-marathon pace 0.5 mile easy 1 mile @ 10K pace 1 mile easy	Core Strength 3 sets	X-Train 1 hour

Week #	Sunday	Monday	Tuesday	Wednesday	Thursday	Friday	Saturday
18	Marathon-Pace Run 6 miles easy + 4 × (2 miles @ marathon pace − 5 sec./mile, 1 mile @ marathon pace + 30 sec./mile)	Core Strength 3 sets	Specific-Endurance Intervals 1 mile easy 5 × 2K @ half-marathon pace w/90-sec. active recoveries 1 mile easy + 10 × 10-sec. hill sprint	Core Strength 3 sets	Threshold Run 1 mile easy 3 miles @ marathon pace 0.5 mile easy 2 miles @ half-marathon pace 0.5 mile easy 1 mile @ 10K pace 1 mile easy	Core Strength 3 sets	X-Train 1 hour
19	Marathon-Pace Run 10 miles easy 10 miles @ marathon pace	Core Strength 3 sets	Specific-Endurance Intervals 1 mile easy 6 × 2K @ half-marathon pace w/90-sec. active recoveries 1 mile easy + 6 × 10-sec. hill sprint	Core Strength 3 sets	Threshold Run 1 mile easy 2 miles @ marathon pace 0.5 mile easy 3 miles @ half-marathon pace 0.5 mile easy 1 mile @ 10K pace 1 mile easy	Core Strength 3 sets	X-Train 1 hour
20	Long Run 12 miles easy	Core Strength 2 sets	Specific-Endurance Intervals 1 mile easy 2 × 2 miles @ half-marathon pace w/2-min. active recovery 1 mile easy + 4 × 10-sec. hill sprint	Core Strength 1 set	Threshold Run 1 mile easy 2 miles @ marathon pace 1 mile easy	Core Strength 1 set	Easy Run 2 miles + 4 × 100m strides

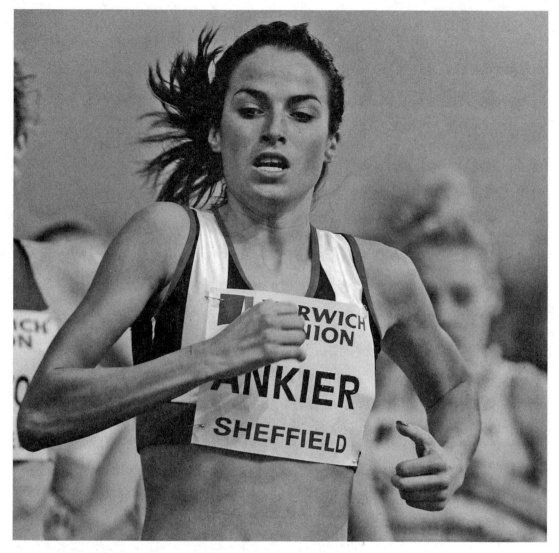

Jo Ankier © Michael Steele, Getty Images

Runner Profile: Jo Ankier

Jo Ankier is one of Great Britain's top middle-distance runners. She contacted me after her friend Jorge Torres told her about the good results he had achieved through working with me. Jo was not willing to relocate to the United States, and I was only lukewarm about the idea of coaching her via e-mail, but we agreed to try working together long-distance on a trial basis and see how it went.

Jo has a lot of natural speed and started as an 800-meter/1,500-meter specialist, but now her focus is the 3,000-meter steeplechase. To build her aerobic strength, I've concentrated on increasing her total running mileage. This was somewhat challenging initially because Jo worked full-time as a television journalist in London. I worked around this constraint by dividing her daily mileage more evenly between morning and evening runs than I would normally do.

Jo's racing has been erratic since I started working with her. She has had some excellent performances and a few forgettable ones. I believe that the keys to improving Jo's consistency and raising her overall level of performance lie in getting her used to running consistently high mileage and in finding the right balance between group and solo training.

I have found that Jo is one of those runners who thrive on intra-group competition in workouts, and she loses motivation when training alone. When I started working with Jo I pulled her out of her group workouts to give her workouts that I thought would serve her better, but for some runners, the wrong workout in the right group is more beneficial than the right workout run alone.

Look for big things from Jo Ankier in the future, after we figure out her optimal training recipe.

Adaptive Training Plans

12

There are 12 unique training plans in this chapter. None of them will be perfectly suited to your needs, because you are much more individual than these workout schedules are individualized. But, if you're training for a 5K, 10K, half-marathon, or marathon, one of them will suit you well enough to start with. Using the adaptive running principles and methods you have learned in reading this book, you'll have no trouble customizing the most appropriate plan to make it an even better fit for you. And even if one of the plans seems perfect when you first look it over, you'll still have to modify workouts as you go based on how your body responds to the prescribed training. Be sure to use the adaptive running guidelines for training execution discussed in chapter 8 to steer this process.

There are three plans for each of the four popular road-race distances. The 5K plans are 12 weeks long, the 10K plans last 14 weeks, the half-marathon plans are 16 weeks long, and the marathon plans last 20 weeks. At each distance there is a level 1 plan, a level 2 plan, and a level 3 plan. The level 1 plans are low training volume plans for beginners and anyone else who needs or prefers a low running mileage program. The level 2 plans are moderate-volume plans for more experienced and competitive runners. The level 3 plans are high-mileage plans for highly competitive runners.

Most of the information you need to perform the workouts correctly is contained within the schedules. For additional details on how to do easy runs, progression runs, long runs, hill sprints, fartlek runs, cross-training ("X-Train") workouts, and strides, refer to the Workout Key on page 213.

5K Training Plans

The training plans in this section are 12 weeks long and culminate in a 5K peak race.

5K Level 1

The running volume in this plan ranges from four runs and 12 miles in week 1 to six runs and 26 miles in week 10.

Week #	Sunday	Monday	Tuesday	Wednesday	Thursday	Friday	Saturday
1	Long Run 4 miles easy	Easy Run 3 miles + 1 × 8-sec. hill sprint	X-Train or Rest	Easy Run 3 miles	X-Train or Rest	Rest	Easy Run 2 miles + 1 × 8-sec. hill sprint
2	Long Run 5 miles easy	Easy Run 3 miles + 2 × 8-sec. hill sprint	X-Train or Rest	Easy Run 4 miles	X-Train or Rest	Rest	Easy Run 3 miles + 2 × 8-sec. hill sprint
3	Long Run 6 miles easy	Easy Run 3 miles + 3 × 8-sec. hill sprint	X-Train or Rest	Easy Run 4 miles	X-Train or Rest	Rest	Easy Run 3 miles + 3 × 8-sec. hill sprint
4	Progression Run 6 miles, last 10 min. moderate	X-Train or Rest	Fartlek Run 4 miles easy w/8 × 20 sec. @ 3K–1,500m pace	Easy Run 4 miles	X-Train or Rest	Rest	Easy Run 3 miles + 5 × 8-sec. hill sprint
5	Progression Run 6 miles, last 15 min. moderate	X-Train or Rest	Fartlek Run 4 miles easy w/8 × 30 sec. @ 3K–1,500m pace	X-Train or Rest	Easy Run 4 miles + 6 × 8-sec. hill sprint	Rest	Easy Run 4 miles
6	Progression Run 6 miles, last 20 min. moderate	X-Train or Rest	Fartlek Run 5 miles easy w/8 × 40 sec. @ 5K–3K pace	X-Train or Rest	Easy Run 4 miles	Rest	Easy Run 4 miles + 7 × 8-sec. hill sprint
7	Progression Run 6 miles, last 30 min. moderate	X-Train or Rest	Hill Repetitions 1 mile easy 6 × 300m uphill @ 3K effort w/jog-back recoveries 1 mile easy	X-Train or Rest	Easy Run 4 miles	Rest	Easy Run 3 miles + 8 × 8-sec. hill sprint

Week #	Sunday	Monday	Tuesday	Wednesday	Thursday	Friday	Saturday
8	Progression Run 6 miles, last 15 min. hard	X-Train or Rest	Specific-Endurance Intervals 1 mile easy 12 × 400m @ 5K–3K pace w/200m jog recoveries 1 mile easy	X-Train or Rest	Easy Run 4 miles	Rest	Easy Run 3 miles + 9 × 8-sec. hill sprint
9	Progression Run 6 miles, last 20 min. hard	Rest	Hill Repetitions 1 mile easy 8 × 300m uphill @ 3K effort w/jog-back recoveries 1 mile easy	X-Train or Rest	Easy Run 5 miles + 10 × 8-sec. hill sprint	X-Train or Rest	5K race 1 mile easy 5K race or time trial 1 mile easy
10	Long Run 6 miles easy	Easy Run 4 miles + 6 × 10-sec. hill sprint	Specific-Endurance Intervals 1 mile easy 6 × 800m @ 5K pace w/2-min. active recoveries 1 mile easy	Rest	Easy Run 6 miles + 8 × 8-sec. hill sprint	X-Train or Rest	Easy Run 5 miles
11	Progression Run 6 miles, last 20 min. hard	Rest	Specific-Endurance Intervals 1 mile easy 5 × 1K @ 5K pace w/400m jog recoveries 1 mile easy	Rest	Easy Run 5 miles + 8 × 8-sec. hill sprint	X-Train or Rest	Easy Run 4 miles
12	Progression Run 6 miles, last 20 min. hard	Rest	Specific-Endurance Intervals 1 mile easy 1 mile @ 5K–3K pace 5 min. easy 8 × 400m @ 5K pace w/1-min. active recoveries 1 mile easy	Rest	Easy Run 3 miles	Easy Run 2 miles + 3 × 100m strides	5K RACE

5K Level 2						
The running volume in this plan ranges from four runs and 20 miles in week 1 to six runs and roughly 40 miles in week 11.						
Week #	Sunday	Monday	Tuesday	Wednesday	Thursday	Friday	Saturday
---	---	---	---	---	---	---	---
1	Long Run 5 miles easy	Rest	Easy Run 5 miles + 1 × 8-sec. hill sprint	Easy Run 5 miles	X-Train or Rest	Easy Run 5 miles	X-Train or Rest
2	Long Run 5 miles easy	Rest	Easy Run 6 miles + 2 × 8-sec. hill sprint	Easy Run 6 miles	X-Train or Rest	Easy Run 7 miles	X-Train or Rest
3	Long Run 6 miles easy	Easy Run 2 miles	Easy Run 6 miles + 3 × 8-sec. hill sprint	Easy Run 6 miles	X-Train or Rest	Fartlek Run 6 miles easy + 12 × 10 sec. @ 1,500m pace	X-Train or Rest
4	Long Run 7 miles easy	Easy Run 4 miles	Easy Run 6 miles + 4 × 8-sec. hill sprint	Easy Run 7 miles	X-Train or Rest	Fartlek Run 6 miles easy + 12 × 20 sec. @ 3K–1,500m pace	Rest
5	Long Run 8 miles easy	Rest	Easy Run 6 miles + 5 × 8-sec. hill sprint	Easy Run 7 miles	X-Train or Rest	Fartlek Run 6 miles easy + 12 × 30 sec. @ 3K–1,500m pace	Rest
6	Long Run 9 miles easy	Easy Run 5 miles + 6 × 8-sec. hill sprint	Fartlek Run 2 miles easy 12 × 1 min. @ 5K pace/1 min. easy 2 miles easy	Easy Run 7 miles	Easy Run 6 miles	Threshold Run 2 miles easy 10 min. @ half-marathon pace 2 miles easy	Rest
7	Long Run 8 miles easy	Easy Run 5 miles + 7 × 8-sec. hill sprint	Fartlek Run 2 miles easy 6 min. @ 10K pace 4 min. easy 4 × 1 min. @ 5K pace/1 min. easy 2 miles easy	Easy Run 6 miles	Fartlek Run 2 miles easy 8 × 1 min. @ 5K pace/1 min. easy 2 miles easy	Easy Run 6 miles + 10 × 100m strides	Easy Run 2 miles

Week #	Sunday	Monday	Tuesday	Wednesday	Thursday	Friday	Saturday
8	5K Race 2 miles easy 5K race or time trial 2 miles easy	Rest	Easy Run 6 miles	Easy Run 7 miles + 8 × 8-sec. hill sprint	Easy Run 6 miles	Threshold Run 2 miles easy 4 × 6 min. @ half-marathon pace w/1-min. active recoveries 2 miles easy	Rest
9	Long Run 10 miles easy	Easy Run 4 miles + 8 × 8-sec. hill sprint	Specific-Endurance Intervals 2 miles easy 2 × (8 × 400m @ 5K pace w/1-min. active recoveries), full recovery between sets 2 miles easy	Easy Run 7 miles	Easy Run 4 miles	Threshold Run 2 miles easy 2 × 10 min. @ half-marathon/10K pace w/1-min. active recovery 2 miles easy	Rest
10	Long Run 8 miles easy	Easy Run 4 miles + 6 × 8-sec. hill sprint	Specific-Endurance Intervals 2 miles easy 6 × 800m @ 5K pace w/400m jog recoveries 2 miles easy	Easy Run 7 miles	Easy Run 6 miles	Threshold Run 2 miles easy 4 miles @ half-marathon pace 2 miles easy	Rest
11	Long Run 8 miles easy	Easy Run 4 miles + 4 × 8-sec. hill sprint	Specific-Endurance Intervals 2 miles easy 5 × 1K @ 5K pace w/400m jog recoveries 2 miles easy	Easy Run 7 miles	Easy Run 6 miles	Threshold Run 2 miles easy 2 × 10 min. @ half-marathon/10K pace w/1-min. active recovery 2 miles easy	Rest

Week #	Sunday	Monday	Tuesday	Wednesday	Thursday	Friday	Saturday
12	Long Run 8 miles easy	Easy Run 4 miles + 3 × 8-sec. hill sprint	Specific-Endurance Intervals 2 miles easy 1 mile @ 5K pace 800m easy 4 × 400m @ 3K pace w/200m active recoveries 2 miles easy	Easy Run 3 miles	Easy Run 3 miles	Easy Run 3 miles	5K RACE

5K Level 3

The running volume in this plan ranges from five runs and 27 miles in week 1 to six runs and roughly 52 miles in week 10.

Week #	Sunday	Monday	Tuesday	Wednesday	Thursday	Friday	Saturday
1	Long Run 6 miles easy	Rest	Easy Run 5 miles	Easy Run 6 miles	X-Train or Rest	Easy Run 5 miles + 1 × 8-sec. hill sprint	Easy Run 5 miles
2	Long Run 7 miles easy	Rest	Easy Run 6 miles + 1 × 8-sec. hill sprint	Easy Run 7 miles	X-Train or Rest	Easy Run 6 miles + 2 × 8-sec. hill sprint	Easy Run 5 miles
3	Progression Run 8 miles, last 5 min. moderate	Easy Run 5 miles + 3 × 8-sec. hill sprint	Easy Run 6 miles	Fartlek Run 7 miles easy w/8 × 20 sec. @ 3K–1,500m pace	X-Train or Rest	Easy Run 7 miles + 4 × 8-sec. hill sprint	Easy Run 5 miles
4	Progression Run 9 miles, last 10 min. moderate	Easy Run 5 miles + 5 × 8-sec. hill sprint	Easy Run 6 miles	Fartlek Run 8 miles easy w/8 × 25 sec. @ 3K–1,500m pace	X-Train or Rest	Easy Run 7 miles + 6 × 8-sec. hill sprint	Easy Run 5 miles
5	Progression Run 10 miles, last 15 min. moderate	Easy Run 6 miles + 7 × 8-sec. hill sprint	Easy Run 6 miles	Fartlek Run 8 miles easy w/8 × 30 sec. @ 3K–1,500m pace	X-Train or Rest	Easy Run 8 miles	Easy Run 5 miles

Week #	Sunday	Monday	Tuesday	Wednesday	Thursday	Friday	Saturday
6	Progression Run 11 miles, last 20 min. moderate	Easy Run 5 miles + 8 × 8-sec. hill sprint	Easy Run 6 miles	Fartlek Run 8 miles easy w/8 × 35 sec. @ 3K–1,500m pace	X-Train or Rest	Easy Run 4 miles	5K Race or Time Trial
7	Long Run 10 miles easy	Easy Run 6 miles + 8 × 8-sec. hill sprint	Speed Intervals 2 miles easy 12 × 400m @ 3K pace w/200m jog recoveries 2 miles easy	Easy Run 9 miles	X-Train or Rest	Threshold Run 2 miles easy 3 miles @ half-marathon pace 2 miles easy	Easy Run 6 miles
8	Progression Run 12 miles, last 20 min. moderate	Easy Run 7 miles + 8 × 8-sec. hill sprint	Specific-Endurance Intervals 2 miles easy 6 × 800m @ 5K pace w/400m jog recoveries 2 miles easy	Easy Run 9 miles	X-Train or Rest	Fartlek Run 9 miles easy w/1 min. @ 5K–3K pace	Easy Run 6 miles
9	Long Run 12 miles easy	Easy Run 6 miles + 8 × 8-sec. hill sprint	Specific-Endurance Intervals 2 miles easy 5 × 1K @ 5K pace w/2-min. active recoveries 2 miles easy	Easy Run 10 miles	X-Train or Rest	Threshold Run 2 miles easy 2 × 2 miles @ half-marathon pace w/2-min. active recovery 2 miles easy	Easy Run 5 miles
10	Long Run 12 miles easy	Easy Run 6 miles + 6 × 8-sec. hill sprint	Ladder Intervals 2 miles easy 1,600m, 1,200m, 1,000m, 800m, 400m @ 10K–1,500m pace w/2-min. active recoveries 2 miles easy	Easy Run 10 miles	X-Train or Rest	Threshold Run 2 miles easy 5 miles @ half-marathon/ 10K pace w/2-min. active recovery 2 miles easy	Easy Run 6 miles

Week #	Sunday	Monday	Tuesday	Wednesday	Thursday	Friday	Saturday
11	Long Run 10 miles easy	Easy Run 6 miles + 6 × 8-sec. hill sprint	Ladder Intervals 2 miles easy 2K, 1K, 800m, 400m @ 10K–1,500m pace w/400m jog recoveries 2 miles easy	Easy Run 9 miles	X-Train or Rest	Threshold Run 2 miles easy 2 × 2 miles @ half-marathon pace w/2-min. active recovery 2 miles easy	Easy Run 5 miles
12	Long Run 8 miles easy	Easy Run 5 miles + 6 × 8-sec. hill sprint	Specific-Endurance Intervals 2 miles easy 1,200m @ 5K pace, 6 × 400m @ 5K–3K pace w/1- min. active recoveries 2 miles easy	Easy Run 4 miles	Rest	Easy Run 3 miles + 4 × 100m strides	5K RACE

10K Training Plans

The training plans in this section are 14 weeks long and culminate in a 10K peak race.

10K Level 1							
The running volume in this plan ranges from five runs and 16 miles in week 1 to six runs and 29 miles in week 12.							
Week #	Sunday	Monday	Tuesday	Wednesday	Thursday	Friday	Saturday
1	Long Run 4 miles easy	Easy Run 3 miles + 1 × 8-sec. hill sprint	Rest	Easy Run 4 miles	Easy Run 2 miles	Easy Run 3 miles + 1 × 8-sec. hill sprint	Rest
2	Long Run 5 miles easy	Easy Run 3 miles + 2 × 8-sec. hill sprint	Rest	Easy Run 4 miles	Easy Run 3 miles	Easy Run 3 miles + 2 × 8-sec. hill sprint	Rest
3	Long Run 6 miles easy	Easy Run 3 miles + 3 × 8-sec. hill sprint	Rest	Easy Run 5 miles	Easy Run 3 miles	Easy Run 3 miles + 4 × 8-sec. hill sprint	Rest

Week #	Sunday	Monday	Tuesday	Wednesday	Thursday	Friday	Saturday
4	Progression Run 6 miles, last 10 min. moderate (uphill, if possible)	Easy Run 3 miles + 4 × 8-sec. hill sprint	Rest	Fartlek Run 2 miles easy 4 × 30 sec. @ 1,500m pace, w/2.5-min. active recoveries 2 miles easy	Easy Run 3 miles	Easy Run 3 miles + 4 × 8-sec. hill sprint	Rest
5	Progression Run 7 miles, last 15 min. moderate (uphill, if possible)	Easy Run 3 miles + 5 × 8-sec. hill sprint	Rest	Fartlek Run 2 miles easy 6 × 45 sec. @ 3K pace, w/2:15 active recoveries 2 miles easy	Easy Run 3 miles	Easy Run 3 miles + 5 × 8-sec. hill sprint	Rest
6	Progression Run 7 miles, last 20 min. moderate (uphill, if possible)	Easy Run 3 miles + 6 × 8-sec. hill sprint	Rest	Hill Repetitions 2 miles easy 8 × 300m uphill @ 5K pace, w/jog-back recoveries 1 mile easy	Easy Run 3 miles	Easy Run 4 miles + 6 × 100m strides	Rest
7	Progression Run 7 miles, last 30 min. moderate (uphill, if possible)	Easy Run 3 miles + 7 × 8-sec. hill sprint	Rest	Specific-Endurance Intervals 2 miles easy 15 × 1 min. @ 5K pace/1 min. easy 1 mile easy	Easy Run 3 miles	Easy Run 5 miles + 8 × 100m strides	Rest
8	Progression Run 7 miles, last 20 min. hard (uphill, if possible)	Easy Run 3 miles + 8 × 8-sec. hill sprint	Rest	Hill Repetitions 2 miles easy 8 × 400m uphill @ 5K pace, w/jog-back recoveries 2 miles easy	Rest	Easy Run 3 miles + 3 × 100m strides	5K Race 2 miles easy 5K race or time trial 1 mile easy

Week #	Sunday	Monday	Tuesday	Wednesday	Thursday	Friday	Saturday
9	Long Run 4 miles easy	Easy Run 7 miles	Rest	Specific-Endurance Intervals 2 miles easy 6 × 800m @ 5K pace w/400m jog recoveries 1 mile easy	Easy Run 3 miles	Easy Run 5 miles + 8 × 8-sec. hill sprint	Rest
10	Progression Run 8 miles, last 15 min. moderate	Easy Run 3 miles	Rest	Specific-Endurance Intervals 2 miles easy 8 × 1K @ 10K pace w/400m jog recoveries 1 mile easy	Easy Run 3 miles	Easy Run 5 miles + 8 × 8-sec. hill sprint	Rest
11	Progression Run 8 miles, last 20 min. moderate	Easy Run 3 miles	Rest	Specific-Endurance Intervals 2 miles easy 6 × 1,200m @ 10K pace w/400m jog recoveries 1 mile easy	Easy Run 3 miles	Easy Run 5 miles + 8 × 8-sec. hill sprint	Rest
12	Progression Run 8 miles w/10 min. hard, 5 × 2 min. hard/2 min. easy, 10 min. moderate	Easy Run 3 miles	Rest	Specific-Endurance Intervals 2 miles easy 6 × 1 mile @ 10K pace w/400m jog recoveries 1 mile easy	Easy Run 3 miles	Easy Run 5 miles + 8 × 8-sec. hill sprint	Rest

Week #	Sunday	Monday	Tuesday	Wednesday	Thursday	Friday	Saturday
13	Progression Run 7 miles, last 30 min. moderate	Easy Run 3 miles	Rest	Specific-Endurance Intervals 2 miles easy 2 miles @ 10K pace 5 min. easy 5 × 1K @ 10K pace w/400m jog recoveries 1 mile easy	Easy Run 3 miles	Easy Run 4 miles + 6 × 8-sec. hill sprint	Rest
14	Progression Run 7 miles, last 20 min. hard	Rest	Specific-Endurance Intervals 2 miles easy 1 mile @ 5K–3K pace 5 min. easy 8 × 400m @ 5K pace w/1-min. active recoveries 2 miles easy	Rest	Easy Run 3 miles	Easy Run 3 miles + 3 × 100m strides	10K RACE

10K Level 2

The running volume in this plan ranges from five runs and 26 miles in week 1 to six runs and 48 miles in week 12.

Week #	Sunday	Monday	Tuesday	Wednesday	Thursday	Friday	Saturday
1	Long Run 6 miles easy	Easy Run 5 miles + 1 × 8-sec. hill sprint	Easy Run 4 miles	X-Train or Rest	Easy Run 5 miles + 1 × 8-sec. hill sprint	Easy Run 6 miles	Rest
2	Long Run 7 miles easy	Easy Run 5 miles + 2 × 8-sec. hill sprint	Easy Run 5 miles	X-Train or Rest	Easy Run 5 miles + 2 × 8-sec. hill sprint	Easy Run 6 miles	Rest
3	Progression Run 8 miles, last 20 min. moderate	Easy Run 5 miles + 3 × 8-sec. hill sprint	Easy Run 6 miles	X-Train or Rest	Easy Run 5 miles + 3 × 8-sec. hill sprint	Easy Run 6 miles	Rest

Week #	Sunday	Monday	Tuesday	Wednesday	Thursday	Friday	Saturday
4	Progression Run 9 miles, last 20 min. hard	Easy Run 5 miles + 4 × 8-sec. hill sprint	Fartlek Run 2 miles easy 5 × 30 sec. @ 1,500m pace, w/2.5-min. active recoveries 2 miles easy	Easy Run 2 miles	Easy Run 5 miles + 4 × 8-sec. hill sprint	Easy Run 6 miles	Rest
5	Progression Run 10 miles, last 20 min. moderate	Easy Run 5 miles + 5 × 8-sec. hill sprint	Fartlek Run 2 miles easy 6 × 45 sec. @ 3K pace, w/2-min. active recoveries 2 miles easy	Easy Run 2 miles	Easy Run 5 miles + 5 × 8-sec. hill sprint	Progression Run 6 miles, last 10 min. moderate	Rest
6	Fartlek Run 2 miles easy 4 miles: 1 min. @ 5K pace/1 min. easy 2 miles easy	Easy Run 5 miles + 6 × 8-sec. hill sprint	Fartlek Run 2 miles easy 10 × 1 min. @ 5K pace/1:45 easy 2 miles easy	Easy Run 3 miles	Easy Run 5 miles	Progression Run 7 miles, last 15 min. moderate	Rest
7	Progression Run 12 miles, last 30 min. moderate	Easy Run 5 miles + 7 × 8-sec. hill sprint	Fartlek Run 2 miles easy 12 × 1 min. @ 5K pace/90 sec. easy 2 miles easy	Easy Run 3 miles	Easy Run 5 miles	Progression Run 7 miles, last 20 min. @ marathon pace	Rest
8	Progression Run 10 miles, last 20 min. hard	Easy Run 5 miles + 8 × 8-sec. hill sprint	Fartlek Run 2 miles easy 15 × 1 min. @ 5K pace/1 min. easy 2 miles easy	Rest	Easy Run 5 miles	Easy Run 4 miles + 3 × 100m strides	5K Race 2 miles easy 5K race or time trial 1 mile easy
9	Fartlek Run 2 miles easy 4 miles: 90 sec. @ 5K pace/90 sec. easy 2 miles easy	Easy Run 5 miles + 10 × 8-sec. hill sprint	Specific-Endurance Intervals 2 miles easy 2 × (8 × 400m @ 5K–3K pace w/400m jog recoveries), full recovery between sets 2 miles easy	Easy Run 5 miles	Easy Run 4 miles	Threshold Run 2 miles easy 2 × 10 min. @ marathon/half-marathon pace w/2-min. active recovery 2 miles easy	Rest

Week #	Sunday	Monday	Tuesday	Wednesday	Thursday	Friday	Saturday
10	Progression Run 12 miles, last 20 min. moderate	Easy Run 5 miles + 8 × 10-sec. hill sprint	Specific-Endurance Intervals 2 miles easy 6 × 800m @ 5K pace w/400m jog recoveries 1 mile easy	Easy Run 4 miles	Easy Run 5 miles	Threshold Run 2 miles easy 2 × 15 min. @ half-marathon pace w/1-min. active recovery 2 miles easy	Rest
11	Progression Run 10 miles, last 15 min. hard	Easy Run 5 miles + 10 × 10-sec. hill sprint	Specific-Endurance Intervals 2 miles easy 6 × 1K @ 5K pace w/400m jog recoveries 2 miles easy	Easy Run 6 miles	Easy Run 5 miles	Aerobic Test 2 miles easy 4 miles @ half-marathon heart rate 2 miles easy	Rest
12	Progression Run 12 miles, last 20 min. moderate	Easy Run 5 miles + 10 × 10-sec. hill sprint	Specific-Endurance Intervals 3 miles easy 4 × 1 mile @ 10K–5K pace w/400m jog recoveries 3 miles easy	Easy Run 6 miles	Easy Run 5 miles	Specific-Endurance Intervals 2 miles easy 2 × (8 × 400m @ 5K–3K pace w/1-min. active recoveries), 4 min. recovery between sets 2 miles easy	Rest
13	Progression Run 11 miles, last 10 min. hard	Easy Run 4 miles + 8 × 10-sec. hill sprint	Specific-Endurance Intervals 2 miles easy 4 × 2K @ 10K pace w/3-min. active recoveries 2 miles easy	Easy Run 5 miles	Easy Run 3 miles	Threshold Run 2 miles easy 2 × 10 min. @ half-marathon/ 10K pace w/3-min. active recovery 1 mile easy	Rest

Week #	Sunday	Monday	Tuesday	Wednesday	Thursday	Friday	Saturday
14	Long Run 10 miles easy	Easy Run 5 miles + 5 × 10-sec. hill sprint	Specific-Endurance Intervals 2 miles easy 1 mile @ 5K pace 4 min. easy 8 × 400m @ 5K pace w/1-min. active recoveries 2 miles easy	Easy Run 4 miles	Rest	Easy Run 4 miles + 3 × 100m strides	10K RACE

10K Level 3

The running volume in this plan ranges from six runs and 40 miles in week 1 to seven runs and 62 miles in week 12.

Week #	Sunday	Monday	Tuesday	Wednesday	Thursday	Friday	Saturday
1	Long Run 6 miles easy	Easy Run 5 miles + 1 × 8-sec. hill sprint	Easy Run 6 miles	Easy Run 8 miles	Easy Run 5 miles + 2 × 100m strides	Easy Run 8 miles	Rest
2	Progression Run 8 miles, last 10 min. moderate (uphill, if possible)	Easy Run 6 miles + 2 × 8-sec. hill sprint	Easy Run 7 miles	Easy Run 8 miles	Easy Run 6 miles + 3 × 8-sec. hill sprint	Easy Run 9 miles	Rest
3	Progression Run 9 miles, last 15 min. moderate (uphill, if possible)	Easy Run 5 miles + 3 × 8-sec. hill sprint	Easy Run 8 miles	Easy Run 9 miles	Easy Run 7 miles + 3 × 8-sec. hill sprint	Progression Run 9 miles, last 10 min. moderate	Rest
4	Progression Run 10 miles, last 15 min. moderate	Easy Run 5 miles + 5 × 8-sec. hill sprint	Fartlek Run 2 miles easy 5 miles easy w/20 sec. @ 1,500m pace every 3 min. 1 mile easy	Easy Run 9 miles	Easy Run 7 miles	Progression Run 9 miles, last 15 min. moderate	Rest

Week #	Sunday	Monday	Tuesday	Wednesday	Thursday	Friday	Saturday
5	Progression Run 12 miles, last 20 min. moderate (uphill, if possible)	Easy Run 7 miles + 6 × 100m strides	Fartlek Run 2 miles easy 5 miles easy w/30 sec. @ 1,500m pace every 3 min. 1 mile easy	Easy Run 10 miles	Easy Run 7 miles + 6 × 8-sec. hill sprint	Progression Run 9 miles, last 20 min. moderate	Rest
6	Fartlek Run + Progression 2 miles easy 4 miles: 1 min. @ 5K pace/1 min. easy 1 mile easy 3 miles moderate	Easy Run 6 miles	Hill Repetitions 2 miles easy 8 × 1 min. uphill @ 3K effort w/jog-back recoveries 2 miles easy	Easy Run 9 miles	Easy Run 6 miles + 8 × 8-sec. hill sprint	Aerobic Test 2 miles easy 4 miles half-marathon heart rate 3 miles easy	Rest
7	Progression Run 12 miles, last 25 min. moderate	Easy Run 6 miles	Ladder Intervals 2 miles easy 1 min., 2 min., 3 min., 2 min., 1 min., 2 min., 3 min. @ 5K–1,500m pace w/= duration active recoveries 2 miles easy	Easy Run 9 miles	Easy Run 6 miles + 6 × 8-sec. hill sprint	Threshold Run 2 miles easy 2 × 10 min. @ marathon/half-marathon pace w/2-min. active recovery 2 miles easy	Easy Run 4 miles
8	Progression Run 14 miles, last 15 min. hard	Easy Run 6 miles + 6 × 100m strides	Hill Repetitions 2 miles easy 5 × 2 min. uphill @ 5K–3K effort w/jog-back recoveries 2 miles easy	Easy Run 9 miles	Easy Run 6 miles + 8 × 8-sec. hill sprint	Threshold Run 2 miles easy 2 × 15 min. @ marathon/half-marathon pace w/2-min. active recovery 2 miles easy	Easy Run 5 miles

Week #	Sunday	Monday	Tuesday	Wednesday	Thursday	Friday	Saturday
9	Progression Run 12 miles, last 15 min. hard	Easy Run 7 miles	Specific-Endurance Intervals 2 miles easy 2 × (10 × 400m @ 5K pace w/1-min. active recoveries), full recovery between sets 2 miles easy	Easy Run 10 miles	Easy Run 7 miles + 8 × 8-sec. hill sprint	Threshold Run 2 miles easy 10 min. @ marathon pace 10 min. @ half-marathon pace 10 min. @ half-marathon/10K pace 2 miles easy	Rest
10	Progression Run 14 miles, last 20 min. hard	Easy Run 7 miles	Specific-Endurance Intervals 2 miles easy 8 × 800m @ 10K–5K pace w/2-min. active recoveries 2 miles easy	Easy Run 10 miles	Easy Run 7 miles + 8 × 8-sec. hill sprint	Threshold Run 2 miles easy 2 × 15 min. @ half-marathon pace w/1-min. active recovery 2 miles easy	Easy Run 6 miles
11	Progression Run 12 miles, last 20 min. moderate	Easy Run 5 miles	Specific-Endurance Intervals 2 miles easy 8 × 1K @ 10K pace + 5–10 sec./mile w/80-sec. active recoveries 2 miles easy	Easy Run 10 miles	Easy Run 6 miles + 6 × 8-sec. hill sprint	Aerobic Test 2 miles easy 4 miles @ half-marathon heart rate 2 miles easy	Rest
12	Progression Run 14 miles, last 15 min. hard	Easy Run 7 miles	Specific-Endurance Intervals 2 miles easy 3 × (2K @ 10K pace/1K easy) 2 miles easy	Easy Run 12 miles	Easy Run 8 miles + 6 × 8-sec. hill sprint	Threshold Run 2 miles easy 2 × 15 min. @ half-marathon pace w/1-min. active recovery 2 miles easy	Easy Run 5 miles

Week #	Sunday	Monday	Tuesday	Wednesday	Thursday	Friday	Saturday
13	Progression Run 10 miles, last 20 min. moderate	Easy Run 5 miles	Specific-Endurance Intervals 2 miles easy 4 × 2K @ 10K pace w/3-min. active recoveries 2 miles easy	Easy Run 10 miles	Easy Run 8 miles + 6 × 8-sec. hill sprint	Threshold Run + Speed Intervals 2 miles easy 2 × 10 min. @ half-marathon/ 10K pace w/2-min. active recovery 8 × 200m @ 3K pace w/200m jog recoveries 1 mile easy	Rest
14	Progression Run 10 miles, last 20 min. moderate	Easy Run 6 miles	Specific-Endurance Intervals 2 miles easy 1 mile @ 5K pace 4 min. easy 8 × 400m @ 3K pace w/1-min. active recoveries 2 miles easy	Easy Run 6 miles	Easy Run 4 miles	Easy Run 4 miles + 3 × 100m strides	10K RACE

Half-Marathon Training Plans

The training plans in this section are 16 weeks long and culminate in a half-marathon peak race.

Half-Marathon Level 1							
The running volume in this plan ranges from five runs and 28 miles in week 1 to five runs and 38 miles in week 14.							
Week #	Sunday	Monday	Tuesday	Wednesday	Thursday	Friday	Saturday
1	Long Run 5 miles easy	Easy Run 3 miles + 3 × 8-sec. hill sprint	Easy Run 5 miles	Easy Run 6 miles	X-Train or Rest	Easy Run 6 miles + 3 × 8-sec. hill sprint	X-Train or Rest
2	Long Run 6 miles easy	Easy Run 6 miles + 4 × 8-sec. hill sprint	Easy Run 5 miles	Easy Run 6 miles	X-Train or Rest	Easy Run 5 miles + 4 × 8-sec. hill sprint	X-Train or Rest

Week #	Sunday	Monday	Tuesday	Wednesday	Thursday	Friday	Saturday
3	Long Run 7 miles easy	Easy Run 6 miles + 5 × 8-sec. hill sprint	Fartlek Run 7 miles easy w/6 × 30 sec. @ 10K–3K pace	Rest	Easy Run 4 miles + 5 × 8-sec. hill sprint	Progression Run 6 miles, last 5 min. moderate	Rest
4	Long Run 8 miles easy	Easy Run 6 miles + 6 × 8-sec. hill sprint	Fartlek Run 8 miles easy w/6 × 35 sec. @ 10K–3K pace	Rest	Easy Run 4 miles + 6 × 8-sec. hill sprint	Progression Run 7 miles, last 10 min. moderate	Rest
5	Progression Run 9 miles, last 15 min. moderate (uphill, if possible)	Easy Run 6 miles	Fartlek Run 8 miles easy w/6 × 40 sec. @ 10K–3K pace	Rest	Easy Run 4 miles + 8 × 8-sec. hill sprint	Progression Run 8 miles, last 10 min. moderate	Rest
6	Progression Run 10 miles, last 20 min. moderate (uphill, if possible)	X-Train 30 min.	Hill Repetitions 2 miles easy 6 × 45 sec. uphill @ 3K effort w/jog-back recoveries 2 miles easy	Rest	Easy Run 6 miles + 8 × 8-sec. hill sprint	Progression Run 2 miles easy 3 miles moderate 2 miles easy	Easy Run 4 miles
7	Long Run 11 miles easy	X-Train 30 min.	Ladder Intervals 2 miles easy 1 min., 2 min., 3 min., 2 min., 1 min. @ 5K–1,500m pace w/400m jog recoveries 2 miles easy	Rest	Easy Run 6 miles + 6 × 10-sec. hill sprint	Progression Run 2 miles easy 4 miles moderate 2 miles easy	Easy Run 4 miles
8	Progression Run 12 miles, last 5 min. hard (uphill, if possible)	X-Train 30 min.	Hill Repetitions 2 miles easy 8 × 1 min. uphill @ 5K effort w/jog-back recoveries 2 miles easy	Rest	Easy Run 6 miles + 8 × 10-sec. hill sprint	Progression Run 2 miles easy 4 miles moderate 2 miles easy	Easy Run 4 miles

Week #	Sunday	Monday	Tuesday	Wednesday	Thursday	Friday	Saturday
9	Progression Run 12 miles, last 10 min. hard	Rest	Ladder Intervals 2 miles easy 1 min., 2 min., 3 min., 2 min., 1 min., 2 min., 3 min., 1 min. @ 5K–1,500m pace w/400m jog recoveries 2 miles easy	Easy Run 5 miles	Easy Run 4 miles + 6 × 10-sec. hill sprint	Threshold Run 2 miles easy 2 × 2 miles @ half-marathon/10K pace w/4-min. active recovery 2 miles easy	Rest
10	Long Run 14 miles easy	Rest	Hill Repetitions 2 miles easy 8 × 90 sec. uphill @ 5K effort w/jog-back recoveries 2 miles easy	Easy Run 4 miles	Easy Run 4 miles + 8 × 10-sec. hill sprint	Threshold Run 2 miles easy 5 miles @ goal half-marathon pace 2 miles easy	Easy Run 4 miles
11	Progression Run 12 miles, last 10 min. hard	Rest	Hill Repetitions 2 miles easy 8 × 1 min. uphill @ 5K effort w/jog-back recoveries 2 miles easy	Easy Run 6 miles	Easy Run 4 miles + 6 × 10-sec. hill sprint	Threshold Run 1 mile easy 4 × 1 mile @ 10K pace w/1-min. active recoveries 2 miles easy	Easy Run 4 miles
12	Progression Run 14 miles, last 15 min. moderate	Rest	Hill Repetitions 1 mile easy 4 × 3 min. (1st 90 sec. flat, 2nd 90 sec. uphill) @ 5K effort w/jog-back recoveries 1 mile easy	Easy Run 4 miles	Easy Run 3 miles + 6 × 10-sec. hill sprint	Threshold Run 2 miles easy 6 miles @ current half-marathon pace 1 mile easy	Rest

Week #	Sunday	Monday	Tuesday	Wednesday	Thursday	Friday	Saturday	
13	Progression Run 13 miles, last 20 min. moderate	Rest	Specific-Endurance Intervals 2 miles easy 6 × 800m @ 5K pace w/2-min. active recoveries 1 mile easy	Easy Run 5 miles	Easy Run 3 miles + 6 × 10-sec. hill sprint	Threshold Run 2 miles easy 2 × 3 miles @ half-marathon/10K pace w/30-sec. active recovery 1 mile easy	Rest	
14	Progression Run 14 miles, last 20 min. moderate	Rest	Specific-Endurance Intervals 2 miles easy 5 × 1K @ 5K pace w/90-sec. active recoveries 1 mile easy	Easy Run 3 miles	Easy Run 3 miles + 8 × 10-sec. hill sprint	Threshold Run 2 miles easy 8 miles @ current half-marathon pace 1 mile easy	Rest	
15	Progression Run 12 miles, last 15 min. moderate	X-Train 30 min.	Specific-Endurance Intervals 2 miles easy 2 × 6 min. @ 5K pace w/3-min. active recovery 1 mile easy	Rest	Easy Run 4 miles + 4 × 10-sec. hill sprint	Threshold Run 1 mile easy 2 × 3 miles @ half-marathon/10K pace w/4-min. active recovery 1 mile easy	Easy Run 4 miles	
16	Progression Run 10 miles, last 10 min. moderate	X-Train 30 min.	Specific-Endurance Intervals 1 mile easy 2 × 1 mile @ 10K pace w/3-min. active recovery 1 mile easy	Easy Run 4 miles	Easy Run 4 miles + 2 × 10-sec. hill sprint	Easy Run 4 miles	<u>Sa</u> REST	<u>Su</u> 1/2 MARATHON

The running volume in this plan ranges from six runs and 29 miles in week 1 to six runs and roughly 52 miles in week 14.

Week #	Sunday	Monday	Tuesday	Wednesday	Thursday	Friday	Saturday
1	Long Run 6 miles easy	Easy Run 3 miles + 1 × 8-sec. hill sprint	Easy Run 4 miles	Easy Run 5 miles	Easy Run 4 miles + 1 × 8-sec. hill sprint	Easy Run 5 miles	Rest
2	Long Run 7 miles easy	Easy Run 4 miles + 2 × 8-sec. hill sprint	Easy Run 5 miles	Easy Run 6 miles	Easy Run 5 miles + 2 × 8-sec. hill sprint	Easy Run 7 miles	Rest
3	Progression Run 8 miles, last 10 min. moderate	Easy Run 5 miles + 3 × 8-sec. hill sprint	Easy Run 6 miles	Easy Run 7 miles	Easy Run 6 miles	Progression Run 8 miles, last 10 min. moderate	Rest
4	Progression Run 9 miles, last 15 min. moderate	Easy Run 5 miles + 4 × 8-sec. hill sprint	Progression Run 6 miles, last 10 min. moderate	Easy Run 8 miles	Easy Run 6 miles	Progression Run 8 miles, last 15 min. moderate	Rest
5	Progression Run 8 miles, last 15 min. moderate (uphill, if possible)	Easy Run 5 miles + 5 × 8-sec. hill sprint	Fartlek Run 6 miles easy w/8 × 20 sec. @ 5K–3K pace	Easy Run 7 miles	Easy Run 6 miles	Progression Run 8 miles, last 20 min. moderate	Rest
6	Progression Run 9 miles, last 20 min. moderate (uphill, if possible)	Easy Run 6 miles + 6 × 8-sec. hill sprint	Fartlek Run 8 miles easy w/8 × 30 sec. @ 10K–3K pace	Easy Run 7 miles	Easy Run 6 miles	Threshold Run 2 miles easy 10 min. @ half-marathon pace 5 min. easy 10 min. @ 10K pace 2 miles easy	Rest
7	Progression Run 10 miles, last 20 min. hard (uphill, if possible)	Easy Run 6 miles + 7 × 8-sec. hill sprint	Fartlek Run 8 miles easy w/8 × 40 sec. @ 10K–3K pace	Easy Run 7 miles	Easy Run 6 miles	Threshold Run 2 miles easy 2 × 15 min. @ half-marathon/ 10K pace w/5-min. active recovery 2 miles easy	Rest

Week #	Sunday	Monday	Tuesday	Wednesday	Thursday	Friday	Saturday
8	Progression Run 10 miles, last 30 min. moderate (uphill, if possible)	Easy Run 6 miles + 8 × 8-sec. hill sprint	Fartlek Run 8 miles easy w/8 × 50 sec. @ 10K–3K pace	Easy Run 8 miles	Easy Run 6 miles	Threshold Run 2 miles easy 2 × 15 min. @ half-marathon/10K pace w/2-min. active recovery 2 miles easy	Rest
9	Progression Run 13 miles, last 30 min. hard (uphill, if possible)	Easy Run 6 miles + 9 × 10-sec. hill sprint	Hill Repetitions 2 miles easy 8 × 50 sec. uphill @ 5K effort w/jog-back recoveries 2 miles easy	Easy Run 8 miles	Easy Run 6 miles	Threshold Run 2 miles easy 2 × 15 min. @ half-marathon/10K pace w/1-min. active recovery 2 miles easy	Rest
10	Progression Run 12 miles, last 20 min. moderate	Easy Run 6 miles + 10 × 8-sec. hill sprint	Ladder Intervals 2 miles easy 1 min., 2 min., 3 min., 2 min., 1 min., 2 min., 3 min. @ 5K–1,500m pace w/= duration recoveries 1 mile easy	Easy Run 7 miles	Easy Run 4 miles	Time Trial 2 miles easy 4 miles @ maximum effort 2 miles easy	Rest
11	Fartlek Run + Progression 2 miles easy 4 miles: 1 min. @ 10K pace/1 min. easy 2 miles easy 2 miles hard	Easy Run 6 miles + 8 × 10-sec. hill sprint	Hill Repetitions 2 miles easy 8 × 1 min. uphill @ 5K effort w/jog-back recoveries 1 mile easy	Easy Run 8 miles	Easy Run 6 miles	Threshold Run 2 miles easy 6 miles @ half-marathon pace 2 miles easy	Easy Run 4 miles

Week #	Sunday	Monday	Tuesday	Wednesday	Thursday	Friday	Saturday
12	Progression Run 14 miles, last 20 min. moderate	Easy Run 6 miles + 10 × 10-sec. hill sprint	Fartlek Intervals 2 miles easy 8 × 3 min. @ 10K pace w/2-min. active recoveries 2 miles easy	Easy Run 9 miles	Easy Run 4 miles	Threshold Run 2 miles easy 4 miles @ marathon pace 5 min. easy 4 miles @ half-marathon pace 1 mile easy	Rest
13	Long Fartlek Run 4 miles easy 4 miles: 90 sec. @ half-marathon–10K pace/90 sec. easy 4 miles easy	Easy Run 6 miles + 8 × 10-sec. hill sprint	Specific-Endurance Intervals 2 miles easy 5 × 1 mile @ 10K pace w/3-min. active recoveries 2 miles easy	Easy Run 5 miles	Easy Run 4 miles	Threshold Run 2 miles easy 4 miles @ marathon pace 4 miles @ half-marathon pace 1 mile easy	Rest
14	Long Run 14 miles easy	Easy Run 6 miles + 10 × 10-sec. hill sprint	Specific-Endurance Intervals 2 miles easy 3K @ half-marathon pace, 2K @ 10K pace, 1K @ 5K pace w/3-min. active recoveries 1 mile easy	Easy Run 8 miles	Easy Run 4 miles	Threshold Run 2 miles easy 2 × 4 miles @ half-marathon pace w/5-min. active recovery 1 mile easy	Rest
15	Progression Run 12 miles, last 30 min. moderate	Easy Run 6 miles + 10 × 10-sec. hill sprint	Specific-Endurance Intervals 2 miles easy 5 × 2K @ half-marathon–10K pace w/3-min. active recoveries 2 miles easy	Easy Run 10 miles	Easy Run 4 miles	Threshold Run 2 miles easy 2 × 15 min. @ half-marathon/10K pace w/1-min. active recovery 2 miles easy	Rest

Week #	Sunday	Monday	Tuesday	Wednesday	Thursday	Friday	Saturday	
16	Progression Run 10 miles, last 20 min. moderate	Easy Run 6 miles	Threshold Run 2 miles easy 4 miles @ half-marathon pace 2 miles easy	Easy Run 5 miles	Easy Run 4 miles	Easy Run 4 miles + 4 × 100m strides	Sa R E S T	Su ½ M A R A T H O N

Half-Marathon Level 3

The running volume in this plan ranges from six runs and 32 miles in week 1 to seven runs and 64 miles in week 14.

Week #	Sunday	Monday	Tuesday	Wednesday	Thursday	Friday	Saturday
1	Long Run 6 miles easy	Easy Run 5 miles + 1 × 8-sec. hill sprint	Easy Run 5 miles	Easy Run 6 miles	Easy Run 5 miles + 1 × 8-sec. hill sprint	Rest	Easy Run 5 miles
2	Progression Run 6 miles, last 20 min. moderate	Easy Run 6 miles + 2 × 8-sec. hill sprint	Easy Run 6 miles	Easy Run 7 miles	Easy Run 6 miles + 2 × 8-sec. hill sprint	Rest	Easy Run 5 miles
3	Progression Run 9 miles, last 20 min. moderate (uphill, if possible)	Easy Run 6 miles + 3 × 8-sec. hill sprint	Fartlek Run 7 miles easy w/8 × 20 sec. @ 10K–3K pace	Easy Run 8 miles	Easy Run 6 miles + 3 × 8-sec. hill sprint	Easy Run 7 miles	Rest
4	Progression Run 10 miles, last 20 min. moderate (uphill, if possible)	Easy Run 6 miles + 5 × 8-sec. hill sprint	Fartlek Run 7 miles easy w/8 × 30 sec. @ 10K–3K pace	Easy Run 9 miles	Easy Run 6 miles + 5 × 8-sec. hill sprint	Progression Run 8 miles, last 15 min. moderate	Rest
5	Progression Run 12 miles, last 30 min. moderate (uphill, if possible)	Easy Run 6 miles + 6 × 8-sec. hill sprint	Fartlek Run 7 miles easy w/8 × 45 sec. @ 10K–3K pace	Easy Run 10 miles	Easy Run 6 miles	Progression Run 8 miles, last 20 min. moderate	Rest

Week #	Sunday	Monday	Tuesday	Wednesday	Thursday	Friday	Saturday
6	Fartlek Run 10 miles easy w/10 × 45 sec. @ 10K–3K pace	Easy Run 6 miles + 8 × 8-sec. hill sprint	Fartlek Run 8 miles easy w/8 × 1 min. @ 10K–3K pace	Easy Run 10 miles	Easy Run 6 miles	Time Trial 3 miles easy 4 miles @ maximum effort 2 miles easy	Easy Run 4 miles
7	Progression Run 9 miles, last 15 min. hard (uphill, if possible)	Easy Run 6 miles + 9 × 8-sec. hill sprint	Hill Repetitions 2 miles easy 8 × 1 min. uphill @ 5K effort w/jog-back recoveries 2 miles easy	Easy Run 12 miles	Easy Run 6 miles	Threshold Run 2 miles easy 2 × 15 min. @ half-marathon/ 10K pace w/1-min. active recovery 2 miles easy	Easy Run 6 miles
8	Progression Run 10 miles, last 20 min. hard (uphill, if possible)	Easy Run 6 miles + 10 × 8-sec. hill sprint	Fartlek Run 3 miles easy 15 × 1 min. @ 5K pace/1 min. easy 3 miles easy	Easy Run 10 miles	Easy Run 6 miles	Threshold Run 2 miles easy 6 miles @ half-marathon pace 2 miles easy	Easy Run 4 miles
9	Fartlek Run + Progression 4 miles easy 15 × 1 min. @ 5K pace/1 min. easy 2 miles easy 2 miles hard	Easy Run 6 miles + 8 × 10-sec. hill sprint	Hill Repetitions 3 miles easy 8 × 1 min. uphill @ 5K effort w/jog-back recoveries 3 miles easy	Easy Run 10 miles	Easy Run 6 miles	Threshold Run 2 miles easy 2 × 15 min. @ half-marathon/ 10K pace w/5-min. active recovery 2 miles easy	Easy Run 6 miles
10	Progression Run 12 miles, last 20 min. moderate	Easy Run 8 miles + 8 × 10-sec. hill sprint	Ladder Intervals 3 miles easy 1 min., 2 min., 3 min., 2 min., 1 min., 2 min., 3 min. @ 5K–1,500m pace w/400m jog recoveries 3 miles easy	Easy Run 12 miles	Easy Run 8 miles	Threshold Run 2 miles easy 5 miles @ goal half-marathon pace 2 miles easy	Easy Run 7 miles

Week #	Sunday	Monday	Tuesday	Wednesday	Thursday	Friday	Saturday
11	Progression Run 13 miles, last 20 min. hard	Easy Run 6 miles + 8 × 10-sec. hill sprint	Hill Repetitions 3 miles easy 6 × 2 min. uphill @ 5K effort w/jog-back recoveries 3 miles easy	Easy Run 10 miles	Easy Run 6 miles	Time Trial 3 miles easy 4 miles @ maximum effort 2 miles easy	Easy Run 6 miles
12	Fartlek Intervals 4 miles easy 15 × 90 sec. @ 10K pace/90 sec. easy 4 miles easy	Easy Run 8 miles + 10 × 10-sec. hill sprint	Fartlek Run 2 miles easy 8 × 3 min. @ 10K pace w/2-min. active recoveries 2 miles easy	Easy Run 12 miles	Easy Run 6 miles	Threshold Run 3 miles easy 6 miles @ half-marathon pace 3 miles easy	Easy Run 8 miles
13	Long Run 12 miles easy	Easy Run 6 miles + 10 × 10-sec. hill sprint	Specific-Endurance Intervals 2 miles easy 4 × 1 mile @ 10K pace w/3-min. active recoveries 2 miles easy	Easy Run 12 miles	Easy Run 6 miles	Threshold Run 2 miles easy 3 × 10 min. @ half-marathon/ 10K pace w/2-min. active recoveries 2 miles easy	Easy Run 4 miles
14	Progression Run 15 miles, last 15 min. hard	Easy Run 6 miles + 10 × 10-sec. hill sprint	Specific-Endurance Intervals 2 miles easy 5 × 1K @ 5K pace w/90-sec. active recoveries 1 mile easy	Easy Run 12 miles	Easy Run 6 miles	Aerobic Test 3 miles easy 10K @ half-marathon heart rate 3 miles easy	Easy Run 6 miles
15	Progression Run 13 miles, last 15–20 min. hard	Easy Run 6 miles + 8 × 10-sec. hill sprint	Specific-Endurance Intervals 2 miles easy 5 × 2K @ 10K pace w/3-min. active recoveries 2 miles easy	Easy Run 10 miles	Easy Run 6 miles	Threshold Run 2 miles easy 2 × 15 min. @ half-marathon/ 10K pace w/1-min. active recovery 2 miles easy	Easy Run 4 miles

Week #	Sunday	Monday	Tuesday	Wednesday	Thursday	Friday	Saturday	
16	Long Run 12 miles easy	Easy Run 6 miles + 6 × 10-sec. hill sprint	Specific-Endurance Intervals 3 miles easy 3 × 1 mile @ 10K pace w/3-min. active recoveries 3 miles easy	Easy Run 6 miles	Rest	Easy Run 4 miles + 4 × 100m strides	Sa REST	Su ½ MARATHON

Marathon Training Plans

The training plans in this section are 20 weeks long and culminate in a marathon peak race.

Marathon Level 1

The running volume in this plan ranges from four runs and 15 miles in week 1 to five runs and 50 miles in week 17.

Week #	Sunday	Monday	Tuesday	Wednesday	Thursday	Friday	Saturday
1	Long Run 3 miles easy	X-Train or Rest	Easy Run 3 miles + 1 × 8-sec. hill sprint	Easy Run 6 miles	X-Train or Rest	Easy Run 3 miles + 1 × 8-sec. hill sprint	Rest
2	Long Run 4 miles easy	X-Train or Rest	Easy Run 4 miles + 2 × 8-sec. hill sprint	Easy Run 6 miles	X-Train or Rest	Easy Run 4 miles + 1 × 8-sec. hill sprint	Rest
3	Progression Run 5 miles, last 10 min. moderate	X-Train or Rest	Easy Run 4 miles + 2 × 8-sec. hill sprint	Easy Run 6 miles	X-Train or Rest	Easy Run 5 miles + 2 × 8-sec. hill sprint	Rest
4	Progression Run 6 miles, last 10 min. moderate (uphill, if possible)	X-Train or Rest	Easy Run 5 miles + 3 × 8-sec. hill sprint	Fartlek Run 7 miles w/6 × 30 sec. @ 10K–3K pace	X-Train or Rest	Easy Run 5 miles + 3 × 8-sec. hill sprint	Rest

Week #	Sunday	Monday	Tuesday	Wednesday	Thursday	Friday	Saturday
5	Progression Run 7 miles, last 20 min. moderate (uphill, if possible)	X-Train or Rest	Easy Run 5 miles + 4 × 8-sec. hill sprint	Fartlek Run 8 miles w/6 × 40 sec. @ 10K–3K pace	X-Train or Rest	Easy Run 7 miles + 4 × 8-sec. hill sprint	Rest
6	Progression Run 7 miles, last 20 min. moderate (uphill, if possible)	Rest	Easy Run 3 miles + 4 × 8-sec. hill sprint	Fartlek Run 7 miles w/6 × 50 sec. @ 10K–3K pace	Easy Run 6 miles	Progression Run 8 miles, last 10 min. moderate	Easy Run 4 miles
7	Progression Run 8 miles, last 20 min. moderate (uphill, if possible)	Rest	Easy Run 3 miles + 5 × 8-sec. hill sprint	Easy Run 6 miles	Easy Run 6 miles	Progression Run 8 miles, last 15 min. moderate	Easy Run 4 miles
8	Progression Run 9 miles, last 20 min. moderate (uphill, if possible)	Rest	Easy Run 3 miles + 6 × 8-sec. hill sprint	Fartlek Run 8 miles w/8 × 50 sec. @ 10K–3K pace	Easy Run 6 miles	Progression Run 8 miles, last 20 min. moderate	Easy Run 4 miles
9	Fartlek Run + Progression 3 miles easy 3 miles: 1 min. @ 10K pace/1 min. easy 2 miles easy 2 miles hard	Rest	Threshold Run 2 miles easy 2 × 10 min. @ half-marathon pace w/2-min. active recovery 3 miles easy	Easy Run 9 miles	Easy Run 4 miles + 8 × 8-sec. hill sprint	Progression Run 10 miles, last 20 min. moderate	Easy Run 4 miles
10	Progression Run 11 miles, last 20 min. hard	Rest	Specific-Endurance Intervals 3 miles easy 15 × 1 min. @ 10K pace/1 min. easy 3 miles easy	Easy Run 10 miles	Easy Run 5 miles	Threshold Run 2 miles easy 2 × 15 min. @ half-marathon pace w/3-min. active recovery 2 miles easy	Rest

Week #	Sunday	Monday	Tuesday	Wednesday	Thursday	Friday	Saturday
11	Progression Run 12 miles, last 30 min. hard	Rest	Hill Repetitions 2 miles easy 6 × 1 min. uphill @ 3K effort w/jog-back recoveries 2 miles easy	Easy Run 10 miles	Easy Run 5 miles	Threshold Run 2 miles easy 6 miles @ half-marathon pace 2 miles easy	Rest
12	Long Run 14 miles easy	Rest	Specific-Endurance Intervals 2 miles easy 8 × 800m @ 10K pace w/2-min. active recoveries 2 miles easy	Easy Run 8 miles	Easy Run 5 miles + 8 × 8-sec. hill sprint	Threshold Run 2 miles easy 2 × 15 min. @ half-marathon/ 10K pace w/3-min. active recovery 2 miles easy	Rest
13	Long Run 16 miles easy	Rest	Hill Repetitions 2 miles easy 6 × 2 min. uphill @ 5K effort w/jog-back recoveries 2 miles easy	Easy Run 9 miles	Easy Run 4 miles	Progression Run 2 miles easy 30 min. moderate 2 miles easy	Rest
14	Long Run 14 miles easy	Rest	Specific-Endurance Intervals 2 miles easy 4 × 1 mile @ 10K pace w/3-min. active recoveries 2 miles easy	Easy Run 10 miles	Easy Run 6 miles + 8 × 8-sec. hill sprint	Easy Run 4 miles	Rest
15	Progression Run 18 miles, last 20 min. hard	Rest	Threshold Run 2 miles easy 6 miles @ marathon/ half-marathon pace 2 miles easy	Easy Run 6 miles	Easy Run 4 miles + 10 × 8-sec. hill sprint	Progression Run 7 miles w/ last 10 min. @ marathon pace	Rest

Week #	Sunday	Monday	Tuesday	Wednesday	Thursday	Friday	Saturday
16	Hard Long Run 14 miles @ marathon pace + 20 sec./mile	Rest	Ladder Intervals 2 miles easy 1 min., 2 min., 3 min., 2 min., 1 min., 2 min., 3 min. @ 3K–10K pace w/= duration active recoveries 2 miles easy	Easy Run 8 miles	Easy Run 4 miles + 8 × 10-sec. hill sprint	Progression Run 8 miles, last 15 min. @ marathon pace	Rest
17	Progression Run 22 miles, last 20 min. hard	Rest	Threshold Run 2 miles easy 2 × 15 min. @ half-marathon/10K pace w/1-min. active recovery 2 miles easy	Easy Run 6 miles	Easy Run 4 miles + 8 × 10-sec. hill sprint	Threshold Run 2 miles easy 6 miles @ marathon/half-marathon pace 2 miles easy	Rest
18	Long Run 23 miles easy	Rest	Easy Run 4 miles	Threshold Run + Specific-Endurance Intervals 2 miles easy 4 miles @ marathon/half-marathon pace 3 min. easy 4 × 1 mile @ half-marathon/10K pace w/ 3-min. active recoveries 2 miles easy	Easy Run 4 miles + 8 × 10-sec. hill sprint	Progression Run 6 miles, last 4 miles moderate	Rest

Week #	Sunday	Monday	Tuesday	Wednesday	Thursday	Friday	Saturday	
19	Hard Long Run 2 miles easy 14 miles @ marathon pace + 20 sec./mile 2 miles easy	Easy Run 5 miles	Threshold Run 2 miles easy 2 × 10 min. @ half-marathon pace w/2-min. active recovery 3 miles easy	Rest	Easy Run 4 miles + 10 × 10-sec. hill sprint	Marathon-Pace Run 2 miles easy 8 miles @ marathon pace + 5 sec./mile 1 mile easy	Rest	
20	Hard Long Run 10 miles @ marathon pace + 20 sec./mile	Rest	Marathon-Pace Run 2 miles easy 4 miles @ marathon pace 1 mile easy	Rest	Easy Run 4 miles	Easy Run 4 miles	Sa REST	Su MARATHON

Marathon Level 2							
The running volume in this plan ranges from five runs and 42 miles in week 1 to six runs and 59 miles in week 17.							
Week #	Sunday	Monday	Tuesday	Wednesday	Thursday	Friday	Saturday
1	Long Run 12 miles easy	Easy Run 6 miles + 1 × 8-sec. hill sprint	X-Train or Rest	Progression Run 10 miles, last 5 miles moderate	Easy Run 6 miles + 1 × 8-sec. hill sprint	Progression Run 8 miles, last 10 min. moderate	Rest
2	Long Run 14 miles easy	Easy Run 6 miles + 2 × 8-sec. hill sprint	X-Train or Rest	Progression Run 12 miles, last 6 miles moderate	Easy Run 6 miles + 2 × 8-sec. hill sprint	Progression Run 8 miles, last 10 min. moderate	Rest
3	Long Run 16 miles easy	X-Train or Rest	Fartlek Run 8 miles w/8 × 20 sec. @ 3K pace	Easy Run 10 miles	Easy Run 4 miles + 6 × 8-sec. hill sprint	Progression Run 9 miles, last 15 min. moderate	Rest
4	Progression Run 14 miles, last 20 min. moderate (uphill, if possible)	Easy Run 4 miles	Fartlek Run 10 miles w/8 × 25 sec. @ 3K pace	Easy Run 11 miles	Easy Run 6 miles + 8 × 8-sec. hill sprint	Progression Run 9 miles, last 15 min. moderate	Rest

Week #	Sunday	Monday	Tuesday	Wednesday	Thursday	Friday	Saturday
5	Progression Run 15 miles, last 30 min. moderate (uphill, if possible)	X-Train or Rest	Fartlek Run 10 miles w/8 × 30 sec. @ 5K–3K pace	Easy Run 10 miles	Easy Run 6 miles + 10 × 8-sec. hill sprint	Progression Run 2 miles easy 6 miles moderate 2 miles easy	Rest
6	Long Run 17 miles easy	Easy Run 6 miles	Hill Repetitions 2 miles easy 6 × 1 min. uphill @ 3K effort w/jog-back recoveries 2 miles easy	Progression Run 10 miles, last 6 miles moderate	Easy Run 6 miles + 10 × 8-sec. hill sprint	Easy Run 8 miles	Rest
7	Hard Long Run 1 mile easy 10 miles @ marathon pace + 10–20 sec./mile 1 mile easy	Easy Run 5 miles	Speed Intervals 3 miles easy 15 × 1 min. @ 5K pace/1 min. easy 3 miles easy	Easy Run 10 miles	Easy Run 8 miles + 10 × 8-sec. hill sprint	Threshold Run 2 miles easy 2 × 15 min. @ half-marathon pace w/2-min. active recovery 3 miles easy	Rest
8	Progression Run 16 miles, last 30 min. hard (uphill, if possible)	Easy Run 4 miles	Hill Repetitions 2 miles easy 6 × 2 min. uphill @ 10K effort w/jog-back recoveries 2 miles easy	Progression Run 10 miles, last 8 miles hard	Easy Run 8 miles + 10 × 8-sec. hill sprint	Threshold Run 2 miles easy 5 miles @ half-marathon pace 2 miles easy	Rest
9	Fartlek Run + Progression 6 miles easy 5 miles: 1 min. @ 10K pace/1 min. easy 1 mile easy 2 miles hard	Easy Run 6 miles	Specific-Endurance Intervals 2 miles easy 3 × 1 mile @ 10K–5K pace w/400m jog recoveries 3 miles easy	Easy Run 10 miles	Rest	Easy Run 6 miles	10K Race 2 miles easy 10K race or time trial 2 miles easy

Week #	Sunday	Monday	Tuesday	Wednesday	Thursday	Friday	Saturday
10	Long Run 8 miles easy	Easy Run 7 miles	Easy Run 10 miles	Fartlek Run 10 miles easy w/30 sec. @ 5K pace every 3 min.	Easy Run 8 miles + 10 × 8-sec. hill sprint	Ladder Intervals 2 miles easy 1 min., 2 min., 3 min., 2 min., 1 min., 2 min., 3 min. @ 3K–10K pace w/= duration active recoveries 2 miles easy	Easy Run 8 miles
11	Fartlek Run + Progression 6 miles easy 5 miles: 90 sec. @ 10K pace/90 sec. easy 2 miles easy 3 miles hard	Easy Run 6 miles	Specific-Endurance Intervals 2 miles easy 4 × 1 mile @ 10K pace w/3-min. active recoveries 2 miles easy	Easy Run 12 miles	Easy Run 6 miles + 10 × 8-sec. hill sprint	Progression Run 10 miles, last 15 min. moderate	Rest
12	Long Run 17 miles easy	Rest	Threshold Run 2 miles easy 6 miles @ marathon/half-marathon pace 2 miles easy	Easy Run 9 miles	Easy Run 4 miles	Fartlek Run 10 miles easy w/2 min. @ 10K pace every 5 min.	Rest
13	Hard Long Run 2 miles easy 14 miles @ marathon pace + 10–20 sec./mile 2 miles easy	Easy Run 4 miles	Easy Run 8 miles	Easy Run 12 miles	Easy Run 4 miles + 10 × 8-sec. hill sprint	Threshold Run 3 miles easy 3 × 10 min. @ half-marathon pace w/3-min. active recoveries 3 miles easy	Rest
14	Long Run 20 miles easy	Easy Run 5 miles	Fartlek Run 3 miles easy 8 × 3 min. @ half-marathon pace/2 min. easy 3 miles easy	Easy Run 12 miles	Easy Run 8 miles + 4 × 8-sec. hill sprint	Fartlek Run 4 miles easy w/6 × 20–30 sec. @ 5K–3K pace	Rest

Week #	Sunday	Monday	Tuesday	Wednesday	Thursday	Friday	Saturday
15	Spec Test 2 miles easy 13.1 miles @ marathon goal pace 2 miles easy	Rest	Easy Run 7 miles	Fartlek Run 10 miles easy w/10 × 30 sec. @ 10K–3K pace	Easy Run 4 miles	Progression Run 3 miles easy 6 miles moderate 2 miles easy	Rest
16	Long Run 22 miles easy	Easy Run 5 miles + 10 × 10-sec. hill sprint	Easy Run 8 miles	Fartlek Run 10 miles easy w/3 min. @ 10K pace every 5 min.	Easy Run 4 miles	Moderate Run 10 miles	Rest
17	Hard Long Run 2 miles easy 15 miles @ marathon pace + 10 sec./mi. 3 miles easy	Easy Run 6 miles + 10 × 10-sec. hill sprint	Ladder Intervals 2 miles easy 1 min., 2 min., 3 min., 2 min., 1 min., 2 min., 3 min. @ 3K–10K pace w/= duration jog recoveries 2 miles easy	Easy Run 12 miles	Easy Run 4 miles	Progression Run 9 miles, last 6 miles accelerate from marathon pace + 20 sec./mile to marathon pace	Rest
18	Long Run 23 miles easy	Rest	Threshold Run 2 miles easy 2 × 15 min. @ half-marathon pace w/3-min. active recovery 2 miles easy	Moderate Run 12 miles	Easy Run 5 miles + 8 × 10-sec. hill sprint	Marathon-Pace Run 1 mile easy 8 miles @ marathon pace 1 mile easy	Easy Run 4 miles
19	Hard Long Run 18 miles @ marathon pace + 20–30 sec./mile	Easy Run 4 miles + 8 × 10-sec. hill sprint	Ladder Intervals 2 miles easy 1 min., 2 min., 3 min., 2 min., 1 min., 2 min., 3 min. @ 3K–10K pace w/= duration active recoveries 2 miles easy	Moderate Run 6 miles	Easy Run 4 miles	Marathon-Pace Run 1 mile easy 2 × 4 miles @ marathon pace w/5-min. active recovery 1 mile easy	Rest

Week #	Sunday	Monday	Tuesday	Wednesday	Thursday	Friday	Saturday	
20	Long Run 13 miles easy	Easy Run 7 miles + 6 × 10-sec. hill sprint	Marathon-Pace Run 2 miles easy 4 miles @ marathon pace − 10 sec./mile 3 miles easy	Easy Run 6 miles	Easy Run 5 miles	Easy Run 4 miles	Sa REST	Su MARATHON

Marathon Level 3

The running volume in this plan ranges from seven runs and 56 miles in week 1 to seven runs and roughly 87 miles in week 17.

Week #	Sunday	Monday	Tuesday	Wednesday	Thursday	Friday	Saturday
1	Progression Run 12 miles, last 5 min. moderate (uphill, if possible)	Easy Run 6 miles + 2 × 8-sec. hill sprint	Easy Run 8 miles	Easy Run 10 miles	Easy Run 6 miles + 2 × 8-sec. hill sprint	Progression Run 8 miles, last 5 min. moderate	Easy Run 6 miles
2	Progression Run 14 miles, last 10 min. moderate (uphill, if possible)	Easy Run 6 miles + 4 × 8-sec. hill sprint	Fartlek Run 8 miles easy w/8 × 30 sec. @ 10K–3K pace	Easy Run 11 miles	Easy Run 6 miles + 4 × 8-sec. hill sprint	Progression Run 10 miles, last 10 min. moderate	Easy Run 8 miles
3	Progression Run 15 miles, last 15 min. moderate (uphill, if possible)	Easy Run 8 miles + 5 × 8-sec. hill sprint	Fartlek Run 9 miles easy w/8 × 40 sec. @ 10K–3K pace	Progression Run 11 miles, last 5 miles moderate	Easy Run 8 miles	Progression Run 10 miles: 5 miles easy, 4 miles moderate, 1 mile @ marathon pace	Easy Run 5 miles
4	Progression Run 12 miles, last 20 min. moderate (uphill, if possible)	Easy Run 8 miles + 6 × 8-sec. hill sprint	Fartlek Run 9 miles easy w/8 × 1 min. @ 10K–5K pace	Progression Run 10 miles, last 5 miles moderate	Easy Run 9 miles	Time Trial 2 miles easy 4 miles @ maximum effort 2 miles easy	Easy Run 5 miles

Week #	Sunday	Monday	Tuesday	Wednesday	Thursday	Friday	Saturday
5	Progression Run 14 miles, last 30 min. hard (uphill, if possible)	Easy Run 8 miles + 8 × 8-sec. hill sprint	Fartlek Run 9 miles easy w/8 × 2 min. @ 10K pace	Progression Run 12 miles, last 5 miles moderate	Easy Run 10 miles	Progression Run 3 miles easy 3 miles hard 3 miles easy	Easy Run 6 miles
6	Progression Run 16 miles, last 20 min. hard	Easy Run 8 miles + 10 × 8-sec. hill sprint	Fartlek Run 9 miles easy w/4 × 5 min. @ 10K pace	Progression Run 12 miles, last 6 miles moderate	Easy Run 8 miles	Threshold Run 2 miles easy 2 × 15 min. @ half-marathon pace w/1-min. active recovery 2 miles easy	Easy Run 6 miles
7	Long Fartlek Run 18 miles easy w/12 × 30 sec. @ 10K–3K pace	Easy Run 8 miles + 10 × 10-sec. hill sprint	Specific-Endurance Intervals 2 miles easy 4 × 6 min. @ 10K pace w/3-min. active recoveries 2 miles easy	Easy Run 15 miles	Easy Run 10 miles	Fartlek Run 6 miles easy w/8 × 30 sec. @ 10K pace	Easy Run 6 miles
8	Race: 10K or 15K	Easy Run 10 miles + 10 × 10-sec. hill sprint	Easy Run 10 miles	Easy Run 10 miles	Fartlek Run 10 miles easy w/12 × 30 sec. @ 10K–5K pace	Easy Run 12 miles	Easy Run 8 miles
9	Specific-Endurance Long Run 1 hour easy 15 × 1 min. @ marathon pace/1 min. easy 30 min. easy	Easy Run 8 miles + 10 × 10-sec. hill sprint	Hill Repetitions 4 miles easy 5 × 3 min. uphill @ 5K effort w/jog-back recoveries 2.5 miles easy	Progression Run 12 miles, last 6 miles moderate	Easy Run 10 miles	Marathon-Pace Run 3 miles easy 8 miles @ marathon pace 3 miles easy	Easy Run 5 miles

Week #	Sunday	Monday	Tuesday	Wednesday	Thursday	Friday	Saturday
10	Hard Long Run 18 miles @ 10% off marathon pace	Easy Run 8 miles + 10 × 10-sec. hill sprint	Threshold Run 3 miles easy 15 min. @ marathon pace w/1 min. easy, 15 min. @ marathon/half-marathon pace w/1 min. easy, 15 min. @ half-marathon/10K pace 3 miles easy	Progression Run 12 miles, last 6 miles moderate	Easy Run 10 miles	Hill Repetitions 4 miles easy 5 × 3 min. uphill @ 5K effort w/jog-back recoveries 2.5 miles easy	Easy Run 5 miles
11	Specific-Endurance Long Run 1 hour steady 10 × 9 sec. @ marathon pace/90 sec. easy 30 min. steady	Easy Run 8 miles + 10 × 10-sec. hill sprint	Progression Run 9 miles: 3 miles easy, 3 miles accelerate from marathon pace to 5K pace, 3 miles easy	Easy Run 14 miles	Easy Run 10 miles	Ladder Intervals 3 miles easy 1 min., 2 min., 3 min., 2 min., 1 min., 2 min., 3 min. @ 3K–10K pace w/= duration active recoveries 3 miles easy	Easy Run 5 miles
12	Progression Run 20 miles, last 30 min. moderate	Easy Run 8 miles + 10 × 10-sec. hill sprint	Specific-Endurance Intervals 3 miles easy 2 × (10 × 400m @ 10K–5K pace w/1- min. active recoveries), full recovery between sets 3 miles easy	Easy Run 15 miles	Easy Run 6 miles	Threshold Run 3 miles easy 2 × 10 min. @ half-marathon/10K pace w/2-min. active recovery 3 miles easy	Easy Run 6 miles

Week #	Sunday	Monday	Tuesday	Wednesday	Thursday	Friday	Saturday
13	Long Run 22 miles easy	Easy Run 6 miles + 10 × 10-sec. hill sprint	Specific-Endurance Intervals 3 miles easy 6 × 800m @ 5K pace w/2-min. active recoveries 3 miles easy	Easy Run 12 miles	Easy Run 6 miles	Threshold Run 3 miles easy 3 × 10 min. @ half-marathon/ 10K pace w/4-min. active recoveries 3 miles easy	Easy Run 6 miles
14	Specific-Endurance Long Run 1 hour steady 5 × 3 min. @ marathon pace/3 min. easy 30 min. steady	Easy Run 6 miles + 10 × 10-sec. hill sprint	Specific-Endurance Intervals 3 miles easy 5 × 1K @ 5K pace w/2-min. active recoveries 3 miles easy	Moderate Run 10 miles	Easy Run 8 miles	Threshold Run 2 miles easy 5 miles accelerating from half-marathon to 10K pace 2 miles easy	Rest
15	Progression Run 22 miles, last 11 miles moderate	Easy Run 6 miles + 10 × 10-sec. hill sprint	Moderate Run 10 miles	Specific-Endurance Intervals 3 miles easy 6 × 1 mile @ 10K pace + 5 sec./mile w/3-min. active recoveries 3 miles easy	Easy Run 10 miles	Easy Run 14 miles	Easy Run 10 miles
16	Half-Marathon Race or Time Trial	Easy Run 6 miles + 10 × 10-sec. hill sprint	Easy Run 8 miles	Easy Run 8 miles	Easy Run 12 miles	Specific-Endurance Intervals 3 miles easy 10 × 1K @ half-marathon– 10K pace w/1-min. active recoveries 3 miles easy	Easy Run 6 miles

Week #	Sunday	Monday	Tuesday	Wednesday	Thursday	Friday	Saturday	
17	Long Run 24 miles easy	Easy Run 8 miles + 10 × 10-sec. hill sprint	Progression Run 2 miles easy 6 miles accelerating from marathon pace to half-marathon pace 2 miles easy	Easy Run 14 miles	Easy Run 10 miles	Threshold Run 3 miles easy 4 × 10 min. @ half-marathon pace w/4-min. active recoveries 3 miles easy	Easy Run 7 miles	
18	Hard Long Run 1 mile easy 18 miles @ marathon pace + 20 sec./mile 1 mile easy	Easy Run 10 miles + 10 × 10-sec. hill sprint	Fartlek Run 12 miles w/8 × 2 min. @ half-marathon pace	Progression Run 14 miles, last 7 miles moderate	Progression Run 10 miles, last 5 miles moderate	Marathon-Pace Run 2 miles easy 10 miles @ marathon pace 2 miles easy	AM: Easy Run 5 miles PM: Easy Run 5 miles	
19	Long Run 20 miles steady	Easy Run 6 miles + 10 × 10-sec. hill sprint	Fartlek Run 11 miles w/8 × 2 min. @ half-marathon pace	Progression Run 12 miles, last 6 miles moderate	Easy Run 8 miles	Marathon-Pace Run 2 miles easy 2 × 4 miles @ marathon pace w/5-min. active recovery 2 miles easy	Easy Run 6 miles	
20	Progression Run 14 miles, last 20 min. moderate	Easy Run 8 miles + 4 × 10-sec. hill sprint	Specific-Endurance Intervals 2 miles easy 4 × 2K @ marathon pace to marathon pace − 15 sec./mile 2 miles easy	Easy Run 6 miles	Easy Run 6 miles	Marathon-Pace Run 2 miles easy 2 miles @ marathon pace 1 mile easy	Sa 4 miles easy	Su M A R A T H O N

Index

Page numbers in *italics* refer to illustrations.

running volume, 11, 24, 135
   aerobic capacity and, 54–56
   average weekly, 55–56
   consistency and intensity, 27–29
   fatigue and, 195
   half-marathon distance, 56
   increasing, 28–29, 120, 122, 129, 130
   injuries and, 29, 120, 130, 195
   long-term improvement and, 190–91, 195
   peak-race goals and, 27
   training plan design, 144–47
   world record breakers and, 209

Schwald, Sarah, 47–48, *47*
self-assessment, 118–37
   aerobic fitness and, 174–75, 196–97
   age and, 123–26
   event-specific, 130–33
   injury history and, 129–30
   long-term goals and, 135–36
   motivation and, 136–37
   neuromuscular fitness and, 196–98
   past race performance and, 126–28
   peak race performance and, 193–94
   recent training and, 119–21
   recovery profile and, 133–35
   running experience and, 122, 192–98
   running volume and, 195
   short-term goals and, 119, 128–29
   specific endurance training and, 198
   training balance and, 195–96
   training execution and, 173–76
   tune-up race performance and, 194
self-coaching, 6, 7–9, 118, 169, 192–98, 204–10
sharpening (training) period, 30, 32, 33–35, 53, 55, 58
   for marathon training, 157
   muscle-training progressions, 95–96
   purpose of, 33
   race-pace training, 30, 34–35
   specific-endurance training and, 101, 105, 110, 111, 198
   speed training and, 85
   training plan design and, 148–49
   for 20-week marathon schedule, 164–65
shin splints, 190
short-term goals, 119, 128–29
slow-twitch muscle fibers, 10, 24, 80, 131
Smith, Andy, 202–3, *202*
specific-endurance training, 18–19, 29, 32, 50–51, 81, 85, 99–117, 124, 131, 175, 191, 196
   for 5K distance, 101, 102, 103–8, 133
   for half-marathon distance, 103–6, 109–10, 121, 133

long-term improvement and, 198
   for marathon distance, 102–6, 111–12, 121
   pace levels and, 101
   peak week, 150
   progression of, 103–6
   for 10K distance, 101, 102, 103–6, 108–9, 131–33, 198
   testing fitness for, 112–15
   workouts, 100–103
specificity principle, 31–32
speed, 5
   increasing running, 207, 210
   muscle fibers and, 10
   training, 41, 84–88
speed intervals, 80, 81, 84–86, 101, 102, 104, 107
speed runners, 130–33, 175
sprints, *see* hill sprints
stress fractures, 24, 116, 169
stride, 76–79, 82
strides and drills, 80, 81, 89–90, 158, 213

"tapering," 193–94
10K distance, 51–52, 53, 62, 130, 131, 167
   aerobic support training for, 65–67
   fartlek intervals and, 108–9, 180
   fitness requirements for, 132
   masters runners training plan for, 223–26
   muscle training for, 86, 90–93, 94, 96
   pace levels, 40
   peak training week for, 149–51
   running volume, 56
   self-assessment for, 131
   specific endurance training for, 101, 102, 103–6, 108–9, 131–33, 198
   testing fitness for, 113, 114
   training plans for, 241–50
   tune-up races and, 153–54
3K distance, 40, 51, 171, 189
3,000-meter steeplechase, 203, 233
threshold runs, 19, 41, 53–54, 56–57, 58, 60–62, 101, 104
   5K peak race, 64–65
   half-marathon peak race, 67–69, 109, 110
   marathon peak race, 69–71
   pace levels, 42–43
   10K peak race, 65–67
   training plan design and, 146, 150, 154–55
time goals, 31, 100, 128, 142
Toland, Sarah, 3, *3*
Torres, Edwardo, 116–17, *116,* 169
Torres, Jorge, 116, 138–39, *138,* 232
training:
   adaptive running principles and, 18–22
   aerobic, *see* aerobic-support training

training (*continued*)
altitude, 209
balance in, 195–96
body adaptation to, 14–17, 18–19, 20–21
conventional methods of, 5–6, 12–13, 14–15,
30, 40–41, 42
core-strength, 46, 190
customization of, 5–6, 7, 10–12, 17
experimentation and, 199–20
fundamental period, *see* fundamental
(training) period
high-intensity systems of, 27–28, 29
individual response to, 16–17, 20–21, 44
interruptions, 181, 187–88
introductory period, *see* introductory
(training) period
masters runners, 211–13, 223–31
muscle, *see* muscle training
off-season slacking, 188
pain and, 169, 170, 181, 182, 183, 189
plan duration, 142–44, 148–49
priorities, 121, 122
race-pace, 15, 30, 31–32, 34–35, 51, 59, 60,
107, 121
responsively, 6–7, 169, 192
rest days and, 44–45
running volume, *see* running volume
self-assessment and, 118–37
sharpening period, *see* sharpening (training)
period
specific endurance, 18–19, 29, 32, 50–51, 81,
85, 99–117
specificity principle of, 31–32
"speed," 41, 84–88
"surprises" during, 12, 21
"tapering" and, 193–94
three-period cycles of, 33–35
threshold, *see* threshold runs
youth runners, 211–22
see also adaptive training plans
training execution, 168–83
adaptability and, 168–70
hill sprints and, 170–71
injury or illness and, 181–83
interrupted cycles and, 181, 187–88
multi-workout adjustments and, 173–76
single-workout adjustments and, 170–72
three-week planned progressions and, 176–80
training plan design, 140–65
elements of, 140–41
"filler" running, 158, 169

as ideal scenario, 168–69
"key workouts," 154–57
peak race and goal choices, 141–42
peak week and, 149–52, 173–74
phase-duration and, 142–44, 148–49
phases of, 148–49
recovery weeks, 152–54, 160, 161, 162, 163
running volume and frequency schedule,
144–47
start date and duration, 142–44
tune-up races and, 152–54
20-week marathon schedule, 158–65
training stimulus, 17, 22, 171, 195–96
treadmill, anti-gravity, 169, 182–83
tune-up races, 137, 152–54, 194

VO$_2$max (maximal oxygen uptake), 50, 52, 100

warm-ups, 111, 200
water consumption, 206
Wetmore, Mark, 1, 138–39
workload modulation, 36–40
workouts:
easy to moderate, 38–40
experimentation with, 199–200
high-intensity, 36–37, 38, 39–40
"key," 37, 133–35, 154–57
ladder, 41, 86–87, 88, 104–5, 132
long-run, 63, 64, 65–67, 69–72
mental exercise and, 44
multi-pace, 39–41
multi-workout adjustments, 173–76
nonweekly cycles of, 41–42
progression run, 59, 64–71
race-specific, 31–32, 64–72, 150
recovery cycles and, 133–34
repetition intervals, 86
sharpening, 15, 32, 33–35
single-workout adjustments, 170–72
specific-endurance, 100–103, 106–10,
131–32
speed-interval, 88
tentative scheduling of, 6, 21–22
threshold, *see* threshold runs
training execution and, 168–83
training plan design and, 144–47, 149–52,
154–57
unproductive, 121
world records, 207–9, 212

youth runners, 204, 211–22